MYCOTOXINS

Abouth the Authors

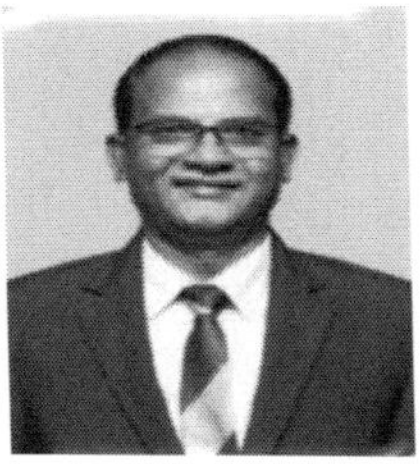

Dr. P. Tensingh Gnanaraj, Ph.D., is currently the Registrar of Tamil Nadu Veterinary and Animal Sciences University, Tamil Nadu, India. He has more than 24 years of experience in the field of Livestock Production and Management.

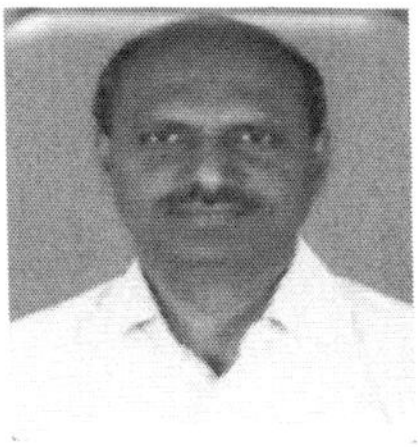

Dr. L. Radhakrishnan, Ph.D., is currently the Professor and Head of Central Feed Technology Unit, a constituent unit of Tamil Nadu Veterinary and Animal Sciences University. He has more than 24 years of experience in the field of Animal Nutrition. He has profound knowledge in the field of feed manufacturing and quality control.

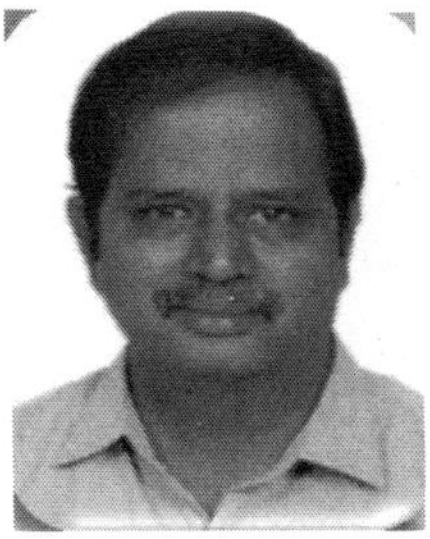

Dr. Ghadevaru Sarathchandra, PhD, is the Dean, Faculty of Basic Sciences, TANUVAS. He is European Registered Toxicologist, FST. He was instrumental in establishing Pharmacovigilance Laboratory for Animal Feed and Food Safety in TANUVAS and in getting ISO/ NABL accreditation to the laboratories of the University.

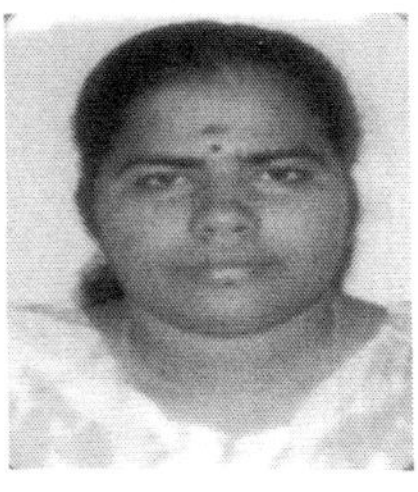

Dr. A. Ruba Nanthini, M.V.Sc, is Assistant Professor working in Central Feed Technology Unit, TANUVAS. She is now in-charge of quality control, production and supply of animal feeds across the state.

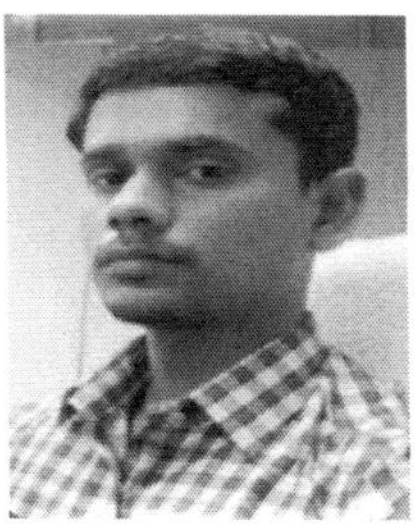

Dr. K. Rajkumar, PhD, is currently working as an Assistant Professor in TANUVAS. He has masters and doctoral degree in Animal Nutrition with specialization in ruminant nutrition.

MYCOTOXINS
A Managemental Guide for Animal Husbandry

P. Tensingh Gnanaraj
L. Radhakrishnan
Ghadevaru Sarathchandra
A. Ruba Nanthini
K. Rajkumar

NEW INDIA PUBLISHING AGENCY
New Delhi-110 034

NEW INDIA PUBLISHING AGENCY
101, Vikas Surya Plaza, CU Block, LSC Market
Pitam Pura, New Delhi – 110 034, India
Email: info@nipabooks.com
Web: www.nipabooks.com

For customer assistance, please contact
Phone: + 91-11-27 34 17 17 Fax: + 91-11- 27 34 16 16
E-Mail: feedbacks@nipabooks.com

ISBN: 978-93-90591-54-1

Composed and Designed by NIPA.

Foreword

India is predominantly an agricultural based country with more than 75% of the population depending on agriculture and agricultural based sectors like animal husbandry. Indian farmers have made enormous contribution to achieve huge increase in food grain production leading to self sufficiency. The country is estimated to have achieved an all time record of 295.67 million tons in the year 2019-20. This is the fourth consecutive year of high production of food grains as per the estimates of Ministry of Agriculture, Government of India. Even though the country has made remarkable progress in the food grain production, several states suffer due to vagaries of weather both due to unpredictable monsoon as well as draught leading to loss of production of food grains causing hardship and consequently economic losses to farmers.

A major portion of food grains produced in rural India gets damaged due to faulty and unscientific storage conditions thus enhancing chances of insect and microbial infestation thereby leading to toxin production. Due to fungal growth, the germination of seed is affected. Also there is discolouration of grain, heating, loss in weight; biochemical changes and toxin production are evident in the stored grain.

Mycotoxins can be extremely harmful to both humans and animals and may be the cause of various medical conditions. Mycotoxins can interfere with the gut integrity by destroying intestinal barrier function, thereby making livestock especially birds becoming vulnerable to invasion of pathogens. They also initiate respiratory diseases in animals and birds. Researchers have also proven the incidence of vaccine failure in farms where there are incidences of mycotoxicosis.

Hence management of mycotoxins is very critical in livestock production for maximizing suitable economic returns. At this juncture, this book is well written to give all basic knowledge about mycotoxins especially to students, research scholars farmers and various other stakeholders. I believe that this book will be very handy for ready reference on mycotoxins.

I congratulate the authors for their sincere efforts in bringing out this book.

Preface

Animal protein sources such as meat, egg and milk are complete proteins as they provide all essential amino acids in highest quality. To provide high quality protein to humans, livestock have to be fed with toxin free quality feedstuffs. Animal feed plays a major role in the global food industry, as it has highest returns to the producer throughout the world. Animal feeds are produced either by livestock farmers themselves locally or feed manufacturing companies. Feeds produced have to be secured and stored in a proper manner to avoid microbial as well as any other biotic agents. Mycotoxins are such naturally occurring toxin produced by the fungal growth. The molds can grow in any of the feed stuffs like maize, other cereals, Groundnut cake and other oil cakes in warm humid climatic conditions.

Mycotoxins can have variety of serious health hazards ranging from mild irritation to deadly cancers in livestock and humans. Addressing the issues related to mycotoxin is the need of the hour. With globalisation of the feed industry and rapid climatic changes, it is very difficult to enumerate the occurrence and presence of the toxin in the feedstuff. These unnoticeable toxin effects may have direct and indirect impact on animal production system. It is very essential to have adequate knowledge about the metabolism, growth and reproduction of various mycotoxins and the toxicological properties of their intermediate products produced during metabolism to neutralize these toxins.

This book gives a basic idea about the mycotoxins, its various types, conditions suitable for their growth, effect of mycotoxins on rumen fermentation, effect of mycotoxin on animal performance, aflatoxin M1 in milk, estimation of mycotoxins, their control measures and application of HACCP in mycotoxin control.

Preventing growth of mycotoxins early with the help of constant monitoring of incoming grains by using various physical, chemical and biological tools during storage will help to avoid higher costs and production losses and thereby increasing profitability to various stakeholders i.e both livestock farmers and feed manufacturers.

Authors

Contents

1

Introduction to Mycotoxins

Mycotoxins are the secondary metabolites produced by moulds, which grow on food and feedstuffs causing pathological or physiological changes to humans and animals. They are toxic to vertebrates in low concentrations. Symptoms depend on the amount of toxin in the feed, the period for which the infested feed is ingested, the nutritional status of the feed and the susceptibility of the animal species. Toxic effects of chronic consumption of mycotoxins in human are carcinogenicity, hepatotoxicity, oestrogenicity, genotoxicity, nephrotoxicity, immunosuppression, reproductive disorders and dermal irritation (Anfossi *et al.,* 2010). The most extensively studied mycotoxins *viz.,* Aflatoxins, ochratoxins, deoxynivalenol (DON, vomitoxin), T-2 toxin, zearalenone, fumoninsins, mycophenolic acid, cyclopiazonic acid and ergot toxins are produced by the moulds *Aspergillus, Fusarium, Pennicillium and Claviceps* (Iqbal *et al.,* 2015).

Aflatoxins

Aflatoxins (AFs) are a major class of mycotoxins produced primarily by *Aspergillus species* including *Aspergillus flavus, Aspergillus parasiticus* and *Aspergillus nom*ius (Creppy, 2002).

Types of Aflatoxins
1. AflatoxinB1 (AFB1)
2. Aflatoxin B2 (AFB2)
3. Aflatoxin G1 (AFG1)
4. Aflatoxin G2 (AFG2)

(Sweeney and Dobson, 1998)

The natural occurrence of aflatoxin has been discovered in many agricultural commodities used as feed ingredients to prepare livestock and poultry feeds. Some of the feed ingredients affected by natural contamination of aflatoxin are maize, oats, sorghum, wheat, barley, groundnut cake, cotton seed oil cake, soybean meal, sunflower oil cake, rapeseed meal and rice bran.

Aflatoxin B1 is generally found in greatest concentration, B2 and G2 in least concentration and G1 at intermediate levels (Salunkhe *et al.,* 1987). Aflatoxin B1 is the most toxic, carcinogenic, teratogenic and mutagenic class of Aflatoxin (Iqbal *et al.,* 2010) and is listed as a group I carcinogen by the International Agency for Research on Cancer (IARC, 2002).

AFB1 and AFB2 are metabolized in the body of animals to produce two other types of aflatoxins namely AFM1 and AFM2, respectively. Another derivative of AFB1 has been detected and is designated as AFM4, which co occurs in certain milk next to AFM1 (Van Egmond, 1989).

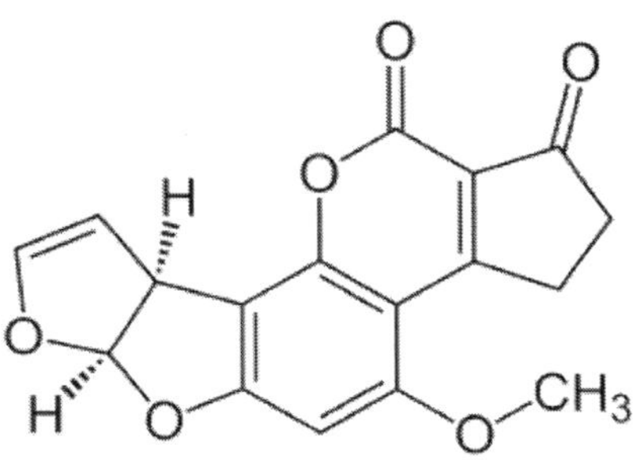

Fig.1.1: Chemical structure of aflatoxin B_1

Metabolism of AFB_1

In the liver, cytochrome P450 system converts AFB-1 into AFM-1 the principal hydroxylated metabolite of AFB-1, found in milk (hence the designation M) of mammals fed upon contaminated feedstuff. Carry-over of AFB-1 as AFM-1 in the milk of dairy cows has been established to range from 0.3 to 6.2% (Veldman *et al.*, 1992) and the metabolic path is shown in figure.1.2. AFM-1 is classified as essentially detoxification product of AFB-1 metabolism as AFM-1 is prevalent even in absence of the metabolic activation of AFB-1 (Neal *et al.,* 1998).

AFB-1 is metabolized in the liver due to the action of the microsomal mixed function oxidase (MFO) enzymes belonging to the super family of CYP450. Upon action of these oxidases, AFB-1 is converted in the reactive 8, 9 - epoxide, existing as two stereoisomers, exo and endo (Neal *et al.,* 1998). The exo-8, 9-epoxide has a high binding affinity toward the DNA, forming the 8, 9-dihydro-8-(N7-guanyl)-9-hydroxy-AFB-1 (AFB-1-N7-Gua) adduct, thus leading to DNA mutations (Verma, 2004).

This epoxide form is involved in other pathways:

(i) Conjugation with glutathione (GSH) catalysed by Glutathione-S-Transferase (GST) with subsequent excretion as AFB-marcapturate; this pathway is vital for the detoxification of AFB-1 as a carcinogen, even if a depletion of GSH could lead to high levels of reactive oxygen species (ROS) causing oxidative damage (Bbosa *et al.,* 2013)

(ii) Enzymatic and non-enzymatic conversion in AFB1-8,9-dihydroxydiol, that can be further converted in the dialdehyde form; aflatoxin dialdehyde can be excreted through urine as dialcohol upon action of aflatoxin aldehyde reductase (AFAR) or can bind proteins, like albumin (Wild and Turner, 2002)

(iii) Binding to other macromolecules like proteins or RNA, causing dysregulation of normal cellular functions and inhibition of proteins, DNA and RNA synthesis (Verma, 2004).

(iv) Microsomal biotransformation of AFB-1 includes hydroxylation of the toxin, leading to the formation of more polar and less toxic metabolites, mainly AFM-1 and Aflatoxin Q1 (AFQ-1).

CYP3A4 is most active isoenzymes of CYP450 and is responsible for the formation of AFB1-exo-8,9-epoxide and of little amount of AFQ1, whereas CYP1A2 leads to both exo- and endo-8,9-epoxide and to the hydroxylated AFM1.

Ochratoxin

Ochratoxin A is a mycotoxin produced by species of the genera Aspergillus and Penicillium, primarily, *Aspergillus ochraceus, Aspergillus melleus* and *Penicillium verrucosum.* Presence of this fungus producing ochratoxin in different food commodities is identified by yellowish-tan color mold growth with *A. ochraceus* to blue–green color mold growth with *Penicillium species* and black color with *A. niger*. Grain and other commodities having a musty odor should be suspect for ochratoxin and mycotoxins.

Ochratoxin A affects the proximal kidney tubules, causing nephropathy in pigs and poultry and is teratogenic in several species of animals. It is a kidney toxin, but in high concentration, it can damage the liver too.

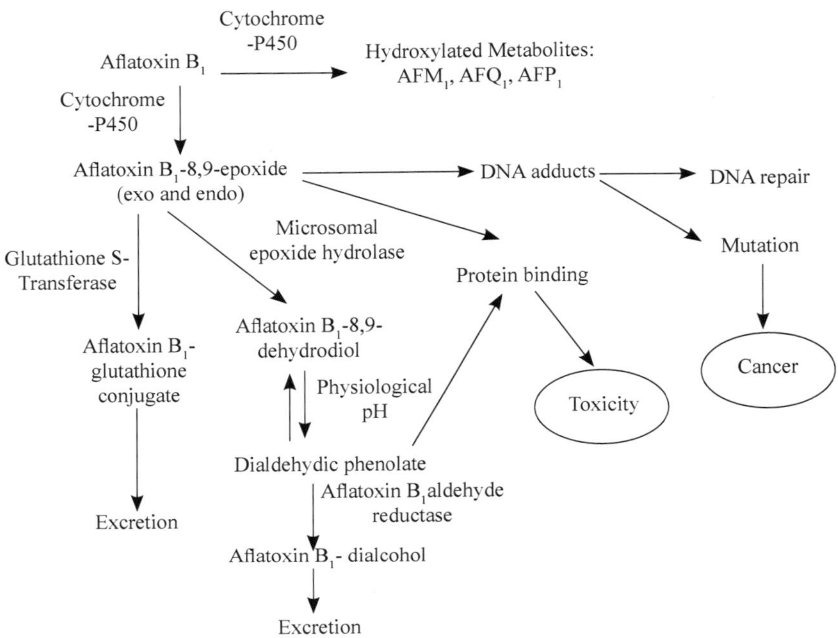

(Adopted from Marchese *et al.,* 2018)

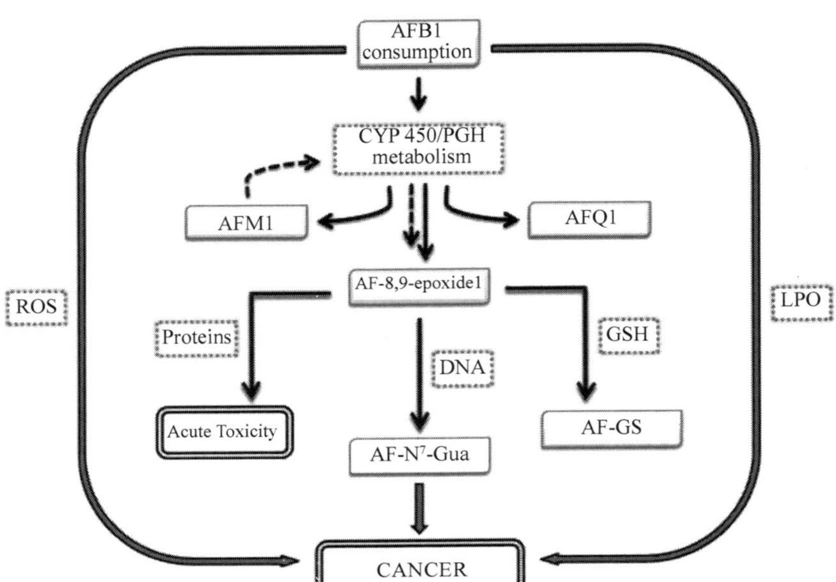

Fig.1.2: Pathways that are involved in metabolism and elimination of aflatoxins in the liver

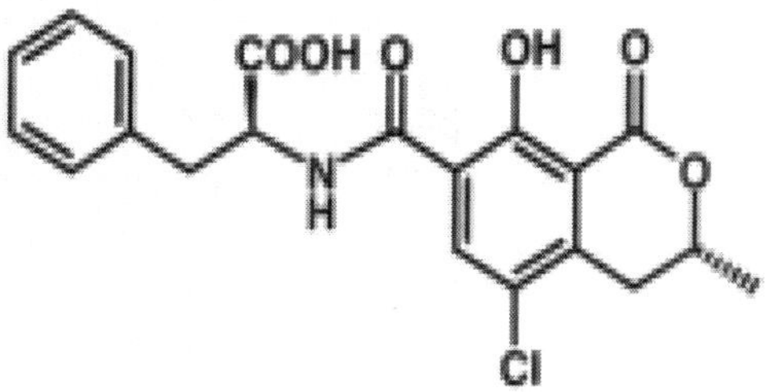

Fig.1.3: Chemical Structure of Ochratoxin

Nephropathy is a kidney disease, often with associated tumors, of humans that is considered by some to be caused by ochratoxin (Pfohl - Leszkowicz *et al.*, 2002). Ochratoxin occurs in a wide variety of commodities such as barley, raisins, soya products and coffee at relatively low levels (CAST, 2003). Its occurrence in house dust and other airborne particulates may be of significance in human disease (Richard *et al.*, 1999; Skaug *et al.*, 2001). Regulations for ochratoxin A are present in the European Community (FAO, 2004).

Table. 1.1: European Union regulation for Ochratoxin

S. No	Product	Concentration (µg / Kg)
1.	Raw cereal grains	5
2.	Dried vine fruit (raisins and sultanas)	10
3.	All products derived from cereals intended for direct human consumption	3

Zearalenone

Zearalenone is an oestrogenic mycotoxin produced by *Fusarium graminearum* or *Fusarium culmorum* (CAST, 2003) and occurs in many agricultural commodities like maize, wheat, barley, sorghum and rye. Grains infected with the above organism may exhibit pink color associated with the production of a pink pigment simultaneously produced with the zearalenone. In wheat, sorghum and maize, zearaleone occurs in pre-harvest grain but in other commodities the surveys are insufficient to determine if zearalenone occurred pre-or postharvest (WHO, 2000). Zearalenone can be formed at relatively cool temperatures and have led to increased levels of this mycotoxin during storage where conditions for fungal growth and mycotoxin formation were favorable.

Pigs are more sensitive to the oestrogenic effects of zearalenone. The consumption of a ration containing 1-5 mg / Kg of zearalenone results in oestrogenic symptoms like swollen and enlarged vulva, vaginal and rectal prolapse, precocious enlargement of the mammary gland, reduced testis size in young males, shrunken ovaries in young females, enlarged, oedematous and tortuous uterus, infertility and abortion. Weak and small litter size piglets have been attributed to the effects of zearalenone when fed to sows during gestation. Consumption of 0.5 to 1.0 μg/g of dietary zearalenone during first half of pregnancy in sows resulted in reduced number of litter size and consumption of zearalenone during late pregnancy does not affect the litter size but resulted in increased number of still borns. Hyperestrogenism in swine occurred with dietary levels of 1.5 to 5 μg/g (Prelusky *et al.*, 1994). Zearalenone appears to bind to estrogen receptors and can result in hormonal changes. Mortalities are not a concern due to zearalenone.

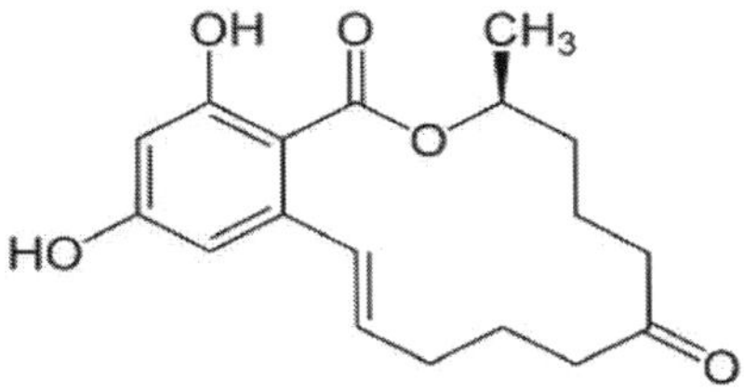

Fig.1.4: Chemical Structure of Zearalenone

Tricothecenes

Several fungal species of the genus Fusarium can produce trichothecenes in agricultural crops and contaminated cereal grains, namely maize, wheat, rye, barley, and rice. All trichothecenes share a tricyclic nucleus named trichothecene (figure.1.5) and usually contain an epoxide at C-12 and C-13, which is essential for toxicity. The total number of naturally occurring trichothecenes known today exceeds 60 (Desjardins *et al.*, 1993) and their chemical structures vary in both the position and the number of hydroxylations and esterifications. According to Marasas *et al.* 1984, six Fusarium species have been well documented worldwide to produce trichothecenes. Two species, *F. sporotrichioides* and *F. poae* produce mainly T-2 toxin and diacetoxyscirpenol. Four species, *F. crookwellense, F. culmorum, F. graminearum,* and *F. sambucinum* produce mainly diacetoxyscirpenol and deoxynivalenol.

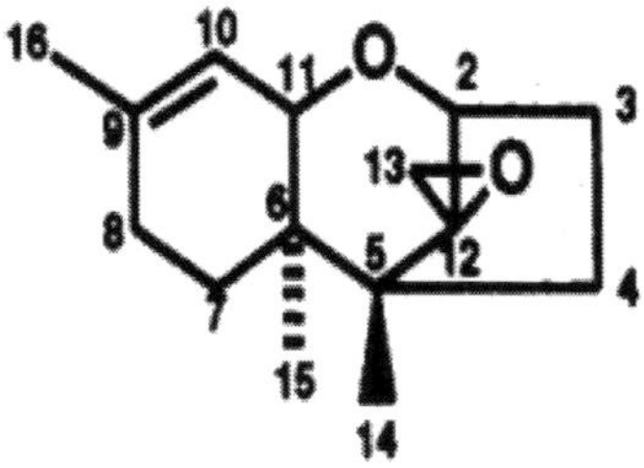

Fig.1.5: Structure of Trichothecene

a) Deoxynivalenol

Deoxynivalenol (figure.1.6) is a Type B nonmacrocyclic trichothecenes and it also known as vomitoxin or DON, is produced principally by *Fusarium graminearum* and in some geographical areas by *F. culmorum* (Richard, 2000). The organisms survive on residue left on the field from the previous season's crop, providing an inoculums source for the new crop. Contamination of the crop occurs when conidia of the organism are windblown to the maize silks. The fungus penetrates the host ear or floret and produces the disease which may be ear rot in maize or head blight in small grains. In maize, the ear rot produced by *F. graminearum* may appear. Wheat heads may appear prematurely and unevenly ripe and the kernels will have a blanched appearance (tombstone kernels) at harvest and may have pink staining present as well. In those commodities where there is pink staining, the disease may be referred to as pink scab.

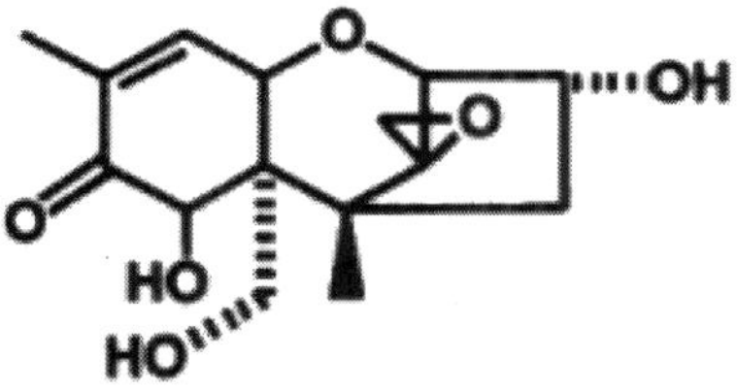

Fig.1.6: Deoxynivalenol

Swine are most severely affected by this toxin and feed intake is reduced; if they do eat it they may vomit. Levels above 1 μg/g are considered potentially harmful to these animals (Richard, 1998). DON is immunosuppressive and may cause kidney problems in animals (Pestka and Bondy, 1994). Humans are thought to exhibit a similar vomition syndrome when consuming DON-contaminated grain (Bhat *et al.*, 1989).

b) T-2 toxin

T-2 toxin (figure.1.7) is a Type A chemical class of non-macrocyclic trichothecenes. This toxin is produced by *F. sporotrichioides*. Some strains of this fungus also produce closely related mycotoxins (HT-2 toxin and diacetoxyscirpenol) belonging to the same chemical class. Usually maize, wheat, barley, oats, rice, rye are reported to contain T-2 toxin (CAST, 2003).

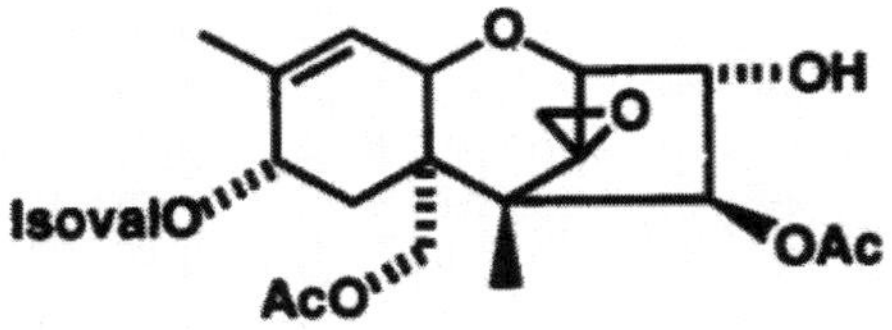

Fig.1.7: T-2 toxin

Natural levels range from near 0 - 10 µg/g with few exceptions up to levels of 40 µg / g visible evidence of the producing fungus may appear on maize as white mold growth which in some instances, may appear pink to reddish, often beginning at the tip of the ear.

The major effect of T-2 toxin and other trichothecenes is that they inhibit protein synthesis. Inhibition of protein synthesis is followed by secondary disruption of DNA and RNA synthesis. Also it affects cells which actively divides like cells lining gastrointestinal tract, skin, lymphoid and erythroid cells. It can decrease antibody levels, immunoglobulins and certain other humoral factors such as cytokines (Niyo *et al.*, 1988; Richard, 1991).

Clinical signs of T-2 toxin are weight loss, bloody diarrhea, dermal necrosis or beak and mouth lesions, hemorrhage and decreased production of milk and eggs. The Type A trichothecenes are more toxic to poultry species than the Type B trichothecenes. Yellow caseous plaques, occurring at the margin of the beak, mucosa of the hard palate, angle of the mouth and tongue, characterize typical oral lesions in poultry. These lesions can occur at dietary levels of 4 mg/kg after one week, 0.4 mg/kg after seven weeks and with 1–4 mg/ kg after three weeks.

Fumonisins

Fumonisins are a group of mycotoxins (FB1, FB2 and FB3) produced by *Fusarium verticillioides* and *F. proliferatum*. Maize, sorghum and rice are most commonly affected grains. The organism producing fumonisin toxin is almost present in every seed and throughout its growth with no symptoms of disease. Grains with insect or bird damage will often contain high levels of toxin. Fumonisins is not a major problem during storage; however, additional care should be taken during harvesting grains without additional kernel damage.

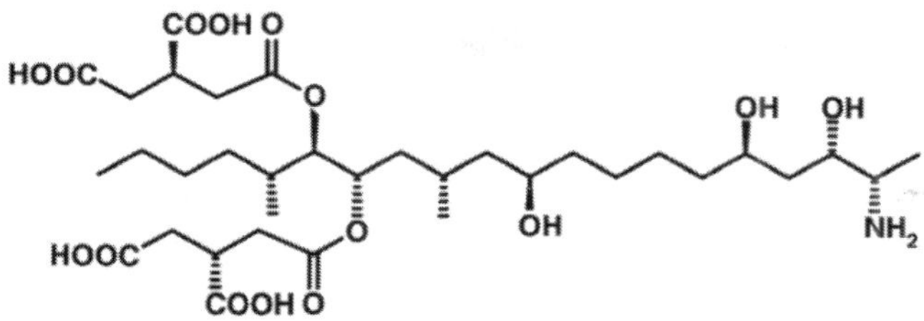

Fig.1.8: Structure of Fumonisin B_1

Fumonisin toxin causes leukoencephalomalacia in horses (Marasas *et al.*, 1988) and lung edema in swine (Colvin and Harrison, 1992). Fumonisin is not carried into the milk and also little absorption in tissues is observed (Richard *et al.*, 1996).

Ergot

Ergotism known popularly as Sanit Antony's fire. Ergot alkaloid produced by *Claviceps species* that affect pasture grasses during the growing season. They are divided into clavine alkaloids (lysergic acid amides) and peptide alkaloids. The fungi, *Neotyphodium coenophialum* produces ergovaline which cause ergot like toxicosis in grazing animals.

Ergotism causes gangrene, central nervous system and gastro intestinal effects in animals. It causes agalactia in swine. The loss of ears and other appendages is common in ergot poisoning.

2

Conditions for Mould Growth and Mycotoxins Production

Various physical, chemical and biological factors interdependently affect the fungal colonization or production of the mycotoxin. Physical factors such as temperature, relative humidity and insect infestations create ideal environment for fungal colonization and mycotoxin production. Stresses such as drought, an increase in temperature, and an increase in relative humidity may selectively alter colonization and metabolism of mycotoxigenic fungi and thus alter mycotoxin production (Russell *et al.*, 1991). Cool and damp weather favours the germination of the sclerotia and thus ergot alkaloid formation in fescue and ryegrass.

Biological factors are categorized into intrinsic factor such as fungal species, strain specificity, strain variation and instability of toxigenic properties. Interaction between the toxigenic fungal species and substrate affect the fungal colonization and mycotoxin production. Some plant species are more susceptible to colonization and some resistant plant species may also get infestation due to favourable environmental conditions.

Moisture and Relative humidity

Moisture content is the most important environmental factors involved in the mould growth and aflatoxin production. Moisture requirement depends upon the temperature as well as nutrient available for growth. When the environmental temperature is optimum for fungal growth, then lowest moisture is enough for mould growth. Similarly, higher moisture requirement is needed for fungal growth at min / max environmental temperature.

According to the moisture requirement, the fungi are divided into three groups:

Hydrophytes – grow at an RH of 90 -100 %

Mesophytes – grow at an RH of 80 - 90 %

Xerophytes – grow at a lower RH limit of 70 %

Relative humidity required for optimum growth of moulds is 80 -90 % and for sporulation is 85 % (Salunkhe *et al.*,1987)

Water activity (a_w)

a_w is a measure of the water available for microbial activity. When the water activity of the grain starts to rises, the xerophilic species will start to develop first. Due to their increased metabolic activity, the moisture content of the grain increases there by making more favorable condition for the mesophytes and hydrophytes. The safest means of preventing fungal growth on grain is to reduce the a_w to below 0.70 equilibrium and to maintain that level throughout the storage period.

Temperature and Time

Based on the temperature needed for the storage fungi to proliferate, the fungi are classified into three groups;

- Psychrophiles
- Mesophiles
- Thermophiles

The minimum, optimum and maximum temperature required for the growth of these groups are given in the table.2.1.

Table.2.1: Minimum, optimum and maximum temperature required for fungus growth

S.No	Fungi group	Minimum temp °C	Optimum temp °C	Max temp °C
1.	Psychrophiles	-5 to 0	10 – 20	25 - 30
2.	Mesophiles	5 -10	20 - 40	40 – 45
3.	Thermophiles	25 – 40	50 – 60	70 - 80

Moulds can grow over a wide range of temperature. The minimum and maximum temperatures are influenced by other growth conditions such as aeration, moisture, nutrients etc. *A. flavus*, a fungus, grows in temperature range between 6 and 46°C, the optimum temperature required is 36 to 38°C (Salunkhe *et al*, 1987). Aflatoxin production is affected by change in temperature range between 5 and 25°C and aflatoxin production stops at temperature below 7.5 and above 40°C.

Optimum time

The optimal time for aflatoxin production by the moulds depends upon the temperature and the moisture content available for growth in the environment.

Environmental temperatures from 25 to 30°C for a period ranging from 7 to 21 days is optimum for aflatoxin production by *A. flavus* and *A. parasiticus*.

Aeration

Fungi are highly aerobic organisms and need a constant supply of oxygen for growth. Oxygen deficiency has a more marked inhibitory effect on the formation of AFB1

Microbial interaction

Microbial competition between fungi for substrate under favourable conditions will reduce the amount of aflatoxin formation. Some of the competing microorganism might restrict or reduce the amount of aflatoxin formation. Sporulation of toxigenic *Fusarium verticillioides* and *F. proliferatum* in maize residues was suppressed by the growth of non- pathogenic *Fusarium species* (Luongo et al., 2005)

Grain condition

Fungi which grows on stored grains leads to severe damage consequently resulting in huge economic losses.

The major types of damage caused by fungi are:

- Initiation of heating processes;
- Reductions in technological qualities;
- Losses in quality;
- Reductions in germination ability;
- Nutritional losses;
- Production of toxic secondary metabolites (mycotoxins).

3

Effect of Mycotoxins On Rumen Fermentation and Nutrient Utilization

The ingestion of mycotoxin-contaminated feedstuffs by animals leads to adverse effect on animal health and the effects are more serious in monogastric animals depending on the species and the susceptibility to toxins within the species. Ruminants are less susceptible to mycotoxins than monogastric animals because of biotransformation of mycotoxins to non-toxic metabolites in rumen by rumen microbiota (Fink-Gremmels, 2008).

The influence of mycotoxins in ruminants in various ways as follows (Upadhaya et al. 2010)

- Dairy animals get exposure to mycotoxins from different feed
- Grazing animals may be exposed to different classes of mycotoxins that occur in pasture grasses (Neotyphodium toxins and ergot alkaloids)
- Potential degradation is saturable and highly dependent on types of forage fed to the animals: changes in feed composition with a high percentage of protein-rich concentrates modify the cleavage capacity of rumen microorganisms
- Some mycotoxins are converted into metabolites that retain or increase their biological activity, such as aflatoxins and zearalenone, respectively
- Antimicrobial activity of the various mycotoxins in the rumen results in impairment of rumen microflora thereby decreasing toxin degrading capacity of the rumen
- High-yielding cows, are more susceptible to metabolic diseases
- Animals in the transition period and in negative energy balance are particularly sensitive to contaminated feeds.

Hence, the maximum tolerable limit of mycotoxins indicated by FDA is 300 ppb for finishing beef cattle instead 20 ppb for poultry. Similarly, the maximum tolerable limit of fumonosins and DON are highest for ruminants and the level is indicated by FDA as 60 and 10 mg / kg respectively. Whereas, for swine, the maximum tolerance limit for fumonosin and DON are 10 and 5 mg / kg, respectively. However, the impact of mycotoxins in ruminant animals depends upon the age, sex, breed, level of the toxin consumed and the immune status of individual animal (Dien and Schatzmayr, 2003).

Sources of mycotoxins in dairy animal feeds

Dairy animals get exposure to mycotoxins by feeding maize by products like dried distillers grain and maize gluten meal. *Fusarium species* are the important mould present in the above said ingredients and produce toxins such as DON, ZEN and FUM. *Aspergillus species* are also prevalent during periods with warmer climate and lower humidity levels suitable for fungal growth.

Dairy animals can get exposure to mycotoxins through roughages whose dry matter is more than 60 % (grass, maize, wheat and grass silage, hay and straw). Important source of mycotoxin in dairy animal is through silage. Silage is favourable media for the growth of Aspergillus, Penicillium, Fusarium and anaerobic and micro aerobic fungal species, such as, *Alternaria, Mucor, Byssochlamys, Geotrichum, Monascus and Scopulariopsis* (Cheli *et al.* 2013). These fungi may produce several important mycotoxins namely gliotoxins, patulin, mycophenolic acid, PR toxin and roquefortines (A, B, C and D). Table.3.1 represents levels of mycotoxin in different type of silages.

Table.3.1: Levels of mycotoxins in different type of silages.

S. No	Toxins type	Maize silage (in ppb)	Grass silages (in ppb)	Grass and Maize silage
1.	Gliotoxins	0 to 878	-	-
2.	Patulin	0.08 (max - 1.21)	-	-
3.	Mycophenolic acid	690 (max – 23000)	2200 (max – 35000)	524 (max – 2630)
4.	Roquefortine C	0.38 (max - 5.71)	100 – 1500	778 (max – 3160)

(Cheli *et al.* 2013).

Effect of aflatoxin in rumen

Various *in vitro* degradation studies with rumen fluid indicated that 42 % degradation of aflatoxin (Engel and Hagemeister 1978) occurs in the rumen. Aflatoxin is degraded in the rumen into aflatoxicol and the remaining portion of aflatoxin that escapes rumen degradation is absorbed in the digestive tract and in the liver by hepatic metabolism which is converted into aflatoxin M- 1 (4-hydroxy metabolite of AFB1). This aflatoxin M -1 is excreted in milk at a transfer rate between 1 % and 6 % (Upadhaya *et al.*, 2010).

Rumen metabolites of aflatoxin retains its biological activity like antimicrobial activity which results in impairment of the function of the rumen flora, followed by a poor feed utilization and reduced weight gain and productivity.

Effect of Trichothecenes in rumen

Trichothecenes produced by *Fusarium* sp such as DON, T-2 toxin and diacetoxyscirpenol are converted into less toxic de-epoxy-trichothecenes in the rumen (Fink-Gremmels, 2008). Hence, ruminants have high tolerance to DON, T-2 toxin and diacetoxyscirpenol. Microbial protein synthesis is reduced by 24 % in rumen fed with *Fusarium* sp contaminated wheat having DON and ZEN toxins (Danicke *et al.*, 2002). Fusarium toxin inhibits the multiplication of cellulolytic bacteria (May *et al.*, 2000) and alters the short chain fatty acids profile and increase the ammonia concentrations which in turn change the microbiota in the rumen (Seeling *et al.*, 2006). *Eubacterium* sp in bovine rumen fluid have the effect of biotransforming the epoxide group of trichothecenes into a diene (Schatzmayr *et al.*, 2006).

Effect of Fusaric acid in rumen

Fusaric acid is also produced by various Fusarium species, occurring in grain feeds especially maize and maize derived foods. Multiplication of *Ruminococcus albus* and *Methanobrevibacter ruminatium* are inhibited by fusaric acids and these species are unable to adapt to the presence of the acid (May *et al.*, 2000).

Effect of Fumonisins in rumen

Fumonisin toxins (Fumonisin B_1) produced by *Fusarium verticilloides* resemble sphingolipids and cause neurotoxity in horses. Fumonisin B_1 resists microbial degradation in rumen. Acute intoxication does not occur under farm condition.

Effect of Zearalenone in rumen

In rumen, Zearalenone is converted into hydroxy metabolite, α – zearalenol, by rumen protozoa which have higher binding affinity to the oestrogen receptors and produce clinical signs of hyperoestrogenism in cows following ingestion of contaminated silage. This component is more active and had lower absorption rate than original molecule zearalenone. (Kennedy *et al.*, 1998). Long term exposure to acute levels of zearalenone produce hyper oestrogenism symptoms in animals (Marczuk *et al.*, 2012).

Effect of Ochratoxin A (OTA) in rumen

Ochratoxin A is produced by *Aspergillus* and *Penicillium species* in the contaminated cereals, grapes, beer, coffee beans and wine (Halasz *et al.*, 2009). Occurrence of Ochratoxicoses in ruminants is rare and amide bond of OTA is hydrolyzed in the rumen by rumen microorganisms into OTA α which has lower toxicity. Animals with well-developed rumen are also affected less by OTA than the pre ruminant calves because degradation of OTA occurs in rumen and convert OTA into less toxic OTA α. (Sreemannarayana *et al.*, 1988).

Mycotoxins such as zearalenone, T-2 toxin, diacetoxyscirpenol and deoxynivalenol are well metabolized in rumen and 90 – 100 % of metabolism is achieved by rumen protozoa (Kiessling *et al.,* 1984). Therefore, rumen protozoa are considered as the most important rumen microorganisms for mycotoxin biodegradations in rumen. However, OTA degradation is carried out by bacterial population of rumen microorganisms (Schatzmayr *et al.,* 2002). *Bacillus licheniformis* in the rumen microbiota is responsible for OTA degradation in Goat (Liu Yang, 2010).

Effect of Patulin in rumen

Patulin, a cyclic lactone produced by species of *Penicillium, Aspergillus* and *Byssochlamys* which occurs in spoiled distillery and apple by products. Patulin has a broad antimicrobial activity against Gram positive bacteria, Gram negative bacteria and protozoa. It has a negative effect on production of volatile fatty acid and protein synthesis in the rumen fluid. (Morgavi *et al.*, 2003). Patulin toxin inhibits rumen cellulolysis as an effect of antimicrobial activity.

Patulin toxin binds covalently to thiol – containing proteins and peptides, including glutathione. Glutathione depletion and subsequent oxidative stress cause neurotoxic symptoms in animals including tremors, ataxia, recumbency and even death. Dietary supplementation of cysteine is used to inactivate the toxin. (Morgavi *et al.*, 2003).

Effect of Ergot alkaloids in rumen

Fungal alkaloids like ergot and ergovaline originating from *Claviceps Sp.* and *Neothyphodium sp* are found in pasture grasses of Northern Europe and in Tall fescue (major pasture grass) of United States. These fungal alkaloids are not inactivated by the rumen microflora and cause Fescue toxicosis. Ergovaline acts as a dopamine receptor agonist and produce clinical symptoms of reduced milk production, low conception rate and loss of body weight.

4

Effect of Mycotoxins on Animal Performance

Mould growth in raw materials or finished feeds result in production of mycotoxins. Mycotoxins are a large group of toxic chemicals causing wide range of pathological and physiological effects in animals. Symptoms depend on the amount of toxin present in the feed, the period for which the feed is ingested, the nutritional status of the feed and the susceptibility of the animal. Feed efficiency, growth rate and production are affected in animals consuming sub-acute doses.

Ruminants are generally considered less susceptible to mycotoxins than monogastric animals because of degradation of mycotoxin in rumen by rumen microorganism. However, certain mycotoxins resist rumen degradation and cause clinical mycotoxicosis. In high yielding dairy animals, during transition period, animals who are in negative energy balance (NEB), low body condition score and decreased resistance to infectious agents cause adverse effects in animal health with exposure of mycotoxins present in animal diet.

Effect of mycotoxin in ruminants

In cattle during metabolism, mycotoxin present in stored or ensiled feeds produce **microbial volatile organic compounds (MVOCs)** which are responsible for mouldy odour, reduced feed intake and increased feeding times. This insufficient feed intake further produces negative energy balance (NEB).

Some of the fungal species like *Aspergillus fumigatus* in silage and hay produce **gliotoxin** which invade tissue and initiates inflammatory process. Further, it causes pulmonary mycosis, abortion or mastitis in cattle. In bulls, it impairs semen quality.

Fungal alkaloids like **ergot and ergovaline** originating from *Claviceps Sp.* and *Neothyphodium sp* are found in pasture grasses and in Tall fescue (major pasture grass). These fungal alkaloids are not inactivated by the rumen microflora and cause **Fescue toxicosis**. Ergovaline acts as a dopamine receptor agonist and produce clinical symptoms of reduced milk production, low conception rate and loss of body weight. Another typical symptom is intolerance to high environmental temperatures, causing a pathological hyperthermia and fat necroses during the summer season as a result of peripheral vasoconstriction caused by ergot alkaloids.

Hyperthermia (summer fescue toxicosis) in cattle is characterized by symptoms of weight loss, salivation and heat stress. Fat necrosis in cattle is characterized by hardened fat resulting in constriction of internal organs, reduced serum cholesterol and elevated serum amylase (Cheeke, 1998). In addition, laminitis and foot gangrene ('fescue foot') suggest the presence of more than one alkaloid in infected tall fescue. Various ergot alkaloids are derivatives of lysergic acid, the latter being the active agent in sleepy grass (*Stipa robusta).*

Festuca grass and rye grass infected with *Neotyphodium lolii* produce **lolitrem B toxin** which act as antagonists to GABAergic neurotransmission causing neurotoxic signs of tremor and ataxia referred as "**Staggers disease**", Ryegrass staggers, Dalli grass staggers, Paspalum staggers and Bermuda grass staggers (Hovermale and Craig, 2001). In sheep, presence of lolitrem B toxin at a level of 2.0 – 2.5 mg /kg with symptoms of shaking with loss of coordination and inability to walk causing staggers.

Rhizoctonia leguminicola fungal species in legume forage plants produce mycotoxin such as **slaframine** which act as partial agonists of cholinergic receptors causing "Slobbers disease" and **swainsonine** metabolite causes a neurotoxic syndrome in livestock with ataxia, depression and tremor (Stegelmeier *et al.*, 1999)

Patulin, a cyclic lactone produced by species of *Penicillium, Aspergillus* and *Byssochlamys* present in spoiled distillery and apple by products, binds to thiol containing protein and peptides, including glutathione and cause neurotoxic symptoms in animals like tremors and ataxia, recumbency and even death. Dietary supplementation of cysteine may be used to inactivate the toxin. (Morgavi *et al.*, 2003).

Aflatoxin intoxication in cattle is characterized by symptoms like poor weight gain, reduced milk production and scouring in calves. Loss of appetite, reduced dry matter intake, decreased rumen motility, liver damage (fatty liver syndrome) and reduced resistance to infection are also often seen in aflatoxin poisoning. The lack of nutrients will interfere with ovarian and uterine functions. This will impair fertility and cause third trimester abortions in cows with the ingestion of 77 μg/ kg of aflatoxin B_1.The concentration of aflatoxin B_1 is likely to produce toxic effects in cattle is 100 μg/ Kg (ppb) and above.

Increased use of aflatoxin contaminated diets in ruminants, induce subclinical, chronic impairment of liver function, and cause hepatic lipidosis following negative energy balance.

Zearalenone and its metabolites like α-zearalenol, bind to oestrogen receptors and induce hyper-estrogenism in animals. Zearalenone causes enlargement of the vulva, edema and swelling of the mammary glands, enlargement of uterus, ovarian cysts, vulvo-vaginitis, atrophy of testicles and ovaries, impaired oocyte maturation and abortion. Zearalenone cause infertility in sheep and cow.

Ochratoxin A is converted into ochratoxin-α in rumen, which is less toxic compared to parent compound. Exposure of cattle to citrinin, a toxin co-occurring with ochratoxin, may cause haemorrhagic syndrome in cattle.

The presence of **T-2 toxin**, one of the prominent type A trichothecenes in feed, result in severe irritation of the upper digestive tract, including hemorrhagic ruminitis, due to its cytotoxic effects in cattle. In the ruminal fluid, T-2 toxin is rapidly degraded into various metabolites, all of which lack significant toxicity. Only a few cases of intoxications in cattle have actually been described (Huszenicza *et al.*, 2000). T-2 toxin cause immunosuppression in cattle by decreasing serum concentration of IgM, IgG and IgA, neutrophil functions and lymphocyte blastogenesis. Immunosuppression by suppressing mitogen induced stimulation of peripheral lymphocytes is also caused by these toxins.

Effect of mycotoxin in pigs

Aflatoxin poisoning in pigs occur at the level of 100 μg/ Kg (ppb) and produce symptoms similar to ruminants like loss of appetite, poor weight gain and scouring in offspring.

Ochratoxin A affects the proximal kidney tubules, causing nephropathy in pigs. On slaughter, kidneys are larger, lighter in colour and firmer than normal. Level of 200 μg/ Kg of ochratoxin A will cause nephropathy in pigs after 3 months.

Pigs are more sensitive to the oestrogenic effects of zearalenone. The consumption of a ration containing 1 -5 mg / Kg of zearalenone results in oestrogenic symptoms like swollen and enlarged vulva, vaginal and rectal prolapse, precocious enlargement of the mammary gland, reduced testis size in young males, shrunken ovaries in young females, enlarged, oedematous and tortuous uterus, infertility and abortion. Weak piglets and small litter size have been attributed to the effects of zearalenone when fed to sows during gestation. Consumption of 0.5 to 1.0 μg/g of dietary zearalenone during first half of pregnancy results in reduced number of litter size and during late pregnancy resulted in increased number of still born. In boars, Zearalenone induced germinal epithelial degeneration and altered sperm formation.

Trichothecenes *viz,* Vomitoxin (Deoxynivalenol), T-2 toxin, Diacetoxyscirpenol (DAS) are large group of toxic compounds produced mainly by the Fusarium fungi. Fusariotoxicosis in pigs cause refusal vomiting syndrome with the symptoms of feed refusal and vomiting. Vomitoxin is the main causative factor of refusal vomiting syndrome and produce these symptoms at the level of 50 -1800 ppb. T-2 toxin and DAS have been associated with haemorrhage in pigs.

Reproductive disorders (e.g. atrophy of the ovaries and uterus, ovarian degeneration, and glandular dysfunction of the endometrium) have been reported in sows exposed to feed contaminated with T-2 toxin

Fumonisin intoxication in pigs, cause pulmonary edema and impairment of cardiac function.

Table 4.1: Effect of toxin in farm animals

S.No	Species affected	Type of mycotoxin	Level of toxin (ppm; mg/ kg)	Effects in animals
1.	Calf	Aflatoxin	0.2 -2.2	Stunting, death, liver damage
2.	Cow	Aflatoxin	2.4	Liver damage
3.	Pigs	Aflatoxin	0.4 – 0.7	Stunting, Liver damage
4.	Laying hens	Aflatoxin	2.5 10 20	Egg production reduced 50 % egg production reduced 100 % egg production reduced
5.	Broiler chicks	Aflatoxin	0.8 1.6	Liver changes detectable Liver changes and weight decrease
6.	Broilers	Aflatoxin	2.5	Body weight reduced
7.	Turkey poults	Aflatoxin	0.125	Growth rate significantly depressed after 12 weeks
8.	Chicks	Ochratoxin A	0.5 1.0 2.0	Decreased egg production Decreased egg size and growth rate Body weight reduced

(Howell. 1982)

Effect of mycotoxin in horses

Mould presence in hay, haylage and straw increase the dust fraction, which contains very high amounts of fungal spores. This causes chronic and recurrent airway disease (RAD) (Laan *et al.*, 2006).

Aflatoxicosis in equines is characterized by depression, lameness and death. Post mortem examinations revealed subcutaneous and enteric hemorrhage, enlarged kidneys, enlarged necrotic livers and myocardial lesions.

Fumonisin B_1 produced by *Fusarium verticilloides* which resembles sphingolipids, cause neurotoxicity in horses leading to leukoencephalomalacia. Symptoms of equine leukoencephalomalacia include ataxia, paresis, apathy hypersensitivity, impaired locomotor function, necrosis of cerebral white matter and lesions in the cerebral cortex.

Effect of mycotoxin in poultry

Chicken are comparatively resistant to aflatoxin compared with pigs and cattle. The level of aflatoxin will begin to produce effects is 500 µg/ Kg and above. However, turkey poults are more sensitive to aflatoxin than are chicken and the level of 100 µg/ Kg of aflatoxin will depress the growth of poults. Aflatoxin increased blood urea nitrogen and decreased serum levels of total protein, albumin, triglycerides and phosphorus.

Poultry are adversely affected by both DON and T-2 toxin and very resistant to the oestrogenic effects of Zearalenone. Feeding of fusarium mycotoxins such as T-2 toxin or DAS have adversely affected chicks with reduced feed intake, body weight gain, buccal- oral ulceration and plaque formation with the dose of 6, 16 and 20 mg / kg of feed in day old, 7 day old chicks and 24 week old hens respectively.

Feeding Ochratoxin A (0.3–1 mg/kg of feed) in broilers reduces glycogenolysis resulting in glycogen accumulation in liver which inturn inhibit protein kinase and decreased feed utilization and teratogenic malformations. Changes in other enzyme activities (e.g. alkaline phosphatase, acid phosphatase, lactate dehydrogenase, and succinate dehydrogenase) resulted in metabolic and cellular respiratory disorders, reduced body weight gain and tissue necrosis.

5

Influence of Aflatoxin M-1 in Milk

Different type of mycotoxins commonly present in different feed and fodder crops are produced by mould during cultivation and storage and are specific to certain region according to climatic and environmental conditions. Most of the toxins produced in crops are consumed when fed to animals. Among the mycotoxins, aflatoxin B-1 is present in highest concentration which enters rumen following ingestion of aflatoxin contaminated feed stuffs. In the rumen, AFB-1 is degraded into aflatoxicol and the remaining portion of the aflatoxin is absorbed in the digestive tract by passive diffusion and metabolized in the liver into aflatoxin M-1 (Kuilman *et al.,* 1998). AFM-1 circulates in the blood as a stable compound until excreted in milk, urine and bile. The following are the sources of AFM-1 contamination in milk and milk products and it occurs through two modes of contamination *viz.,* indirect contamination and direct contamination.

A. Indirect contamination

i. From moulded feed ingredients of cereals and oilseeds

Cereals are normally cultivated, harvested and stored at the livestock farm. During cultivation, Fusarium fungi may infect the cereals in flowering stage. In cereals fungi produces the fusarium toxins deoxynivalenol, nivalenol, zearalenone, fumonisins, HT-2 and T-2 toxins. Avoiding usage of these contaminated cereals in livestock feed manufacturing is very important to lower the adverse effect of mycotoxin ingestion.

Table.5.1: Feed ingredients commonly affected by mycotoxin during storage and in field

S. No	Feed ingredients	Mycotoxins produced in field	Mycotoxin produced in storage
1.	Maize	DON, Fum, Zea	Zea, Afla
2.	Oats	DON, HT- 2, T- 2, NIV	OTA, Cit
3.	Barley	DON, NIV, Zea, HT-2, T-2	OTA, Afla, Cit
4.	Rice	-	Afla, Sterig, OTA
5.	Wheat bran	DON, NIV	OTA
6.	Cotton seed meal	Afla, Tenua	Afla
7.	Groundnut meal	Afla, Zea	Afla, OTA, Cit
8.	Maize grass	Afla	Roq, Pat, Zea
9.	Rye grass	Spor, Lol, Pasp	-
10.	Tall fascue	Ergot	-
11.	Red clover	Slaf	-

Note: Afla –Aflatoxin; Cit – Citrinin; DON – Deoxynivalenol; Fum – Fumonisin; Zea-Zearalenone; NIV – Nivalenol; OTA – Ochratoxin; Tenua – Tenuazoic acid; Roq – Roquefortin; Pat – Patulin; Spor – Sporidesmin; Lol – Lolitrems; Pasp – Paspalitrem; Slaf - Slaframine (Pettersson, 2004)

Maize is commonly harvested at high moisture content. Mycotoxin contamination may be formed, if the final moisture content is above 15 %. Hence, maize should be stored and used for feed preparation at moisture content of around 10 -13%.

Approximately 0.3 to 6.2% of AFB1 in contaminated feed stuff is converted into metabolized AFM1 and excreted in milk, depending on factors such as genetics of the animals, seasonal variation, the milking process and the environmental conditions.

Generally feed ingredients like maize, ground nut cake and milled rice are contaminated with aflatoxin at a level of 5 -35 μg, 5 -35 μg and 0.5–3.5 μg respectively. Analysis report of the maize samples used in feed mill located in Tamil Nadu indicate that 98.40, 17.02, 1.06 and 8.51 % of maize samples were contaminated with Aflatoxin B_1, Aflatoxin B_2, Ochratoxin and citrinin, respectively (Nanthini, *et al.*, 2016). Nearly 57.3 % samples of maize had Aflatoxin B1 above the FDA regulatory level (FDA, 1994) of 20 ppb.

Seasonal influences of aflatoxin contamination in feed stuff

Late monsoon period (Oct to Nov) is more critical period for aflatoxin contamination in feed ingredients. Feed ingredient samples cultivated during late monsoon period and analyzed for aflatoxin contamination have shown higher prevalence of 65.19 %, compared to 25.08, 21.09 and 24.68 % of aflatoxin contamination in winter (Dec- Feb), summer (March to May) and early monsoon (June to Sep) periods respectively.

Aflatoxin enters into the animal through ingestion of contaminated feed ingredients and metabolized by liver into AFM -1 and it's found in milk. Thus, AFM-1 concentration is high in milk samples collected in autumn (El Marnissi *et al.*, 2012); predominantly highest AFM-1 concentration is found in milk samples collected in the rainy season (Diaz and Espitia, 2006).

The animals reared in pasture produces milk with less AFM- 1 than the animals reared in farm fed with stored feed stuffs such as maize by products or cotton seed meal (Diaz and Espitia, 2006). It is a clear indication of transfer of AFB-1 from feed stuff to AFM-1 in milk.

ii. From silage

In ensiling process, maintaining the anaerobic condition is very important for producing good quality silage. If air leakage is found in the silo the mold will be start growing in the silage. In wet silages Fusarium starts growing easily and produces toxin.

Therefore, fodder has to be packed tightly so as to avoid air trapping. Air packets trapped between the crops, lead to invasion of *Penicillium roqueforti*, which will infect the silage and produce roquefortin-C. Also in deteriorated silages, *Aspergillus fumigatus*, *Byssochlamys nivea* and *Paecilliomyces variotti*. A. fumigatus produce gliotoxin and the other two patulin.

iii. From Hay

The following methods are adopted in hay making process; mowing, rapid drying, turning, windrowing, trussing into small heaps and storage. The green crop from the pasture is dried to reduce the moisture content from 70 -90 % to 20 -25 % or less and pressed as bales. During drying the hay gets easily contaminated with soil and rainfall thereby leading to mould growth. Bales pressed out of moist hay easily get contaminated with mould. Fusarium moulds are prevalent in wet crop whereas, *Aspergillus fumigat*us is very common in mould-deteriorated hay.

iv. From Straw

After harvest of the cereals the straw are pressed as bales. The bales are stored without protection from the rain and the straw present in the field will be remoistened by rain and infected by *Stachyobotrys atra*, which produce satratoxin.

v. From contaminated livestock feed

To decrease the level of aflatoxin in milk, feed should be monitored regularly. During feed manufacturing, feed ingredients low in aflatoxin B1 content should be used. There is a linear correlation between AFM1 in milk and AFB1 in feed (Galvano et al., 2001). If feed contains the acceptable level of aflatoxin of 20 μg / kg fed to animal, will result in milk containing less than 0.5 μg / litre of milk i.e. 0.5 ppb (Marth and Steele, 1998).

To prevent mold growth in livestock feed, equipments used in feed preparation should be cleaned thoroughly and the mixer should be free of dust and feed accumulation. If any liquid feed additives are used while preparing feed, the mixer should be cleaned for remnant feed materials.

Fungal growth in feed is prevented by maintaining good sanitation in feed mill and using dry and well ventilated storage structures for packing the prepared livestock feed.

Carryover of AFM-1 in milk

Excretion of AFM1 in milk occurs within 12 to 24 hours of ingestion of AFB1 contaminated feed by the lactating animal. Levels of AFM1 in milk normally peak within 3 to 6 days and decrease to undetectable level. It is reported that carryover rate of AFB1 from ingested feed to AFM1 in milk varies from less than 1.0 to 3.0% (IDF, 1997; Marth and Steele 1998; Van Egmond, 1989) and in some cases to as high as 6.0% (IDF, 1997). Cows who are fed with 500 μg of AFB-1 per day will have a carry-over of 1.63 %. If ingestion of Aflatoxin stops, AFM-1 decreases to undetectable level (0.02 ppb) after 72 hours.

The following factors influence the rate of carry over AFB1 from feed to milk.

- Rate of ingestion
- Feeding regimens
- Rate of digestion
- Health of animal
- Hepatic biotransformation capacity
- Actual milk production

Carryover of AFM-1 in milk is increased in relation to increased milk production and an increase of approximately 0.1 % AFM-1 per kg of milk is obtained (Veldman *et al.*, 1992). The mean carry over value of the cows producing more than 25 liters a day is 2.66 ± 1.24 %. A linear relation exists between quantity of AFB-1 consumed per day and the concentration of AFM-1 in the milk, also the relationship is dependent on milk production. Based on regression equation (Figure.5.1), the AFM-l concentration in the milk is increased by 0.72 ng for every µg of AFB-l consumed, with a correlation coefficient of 0.943.

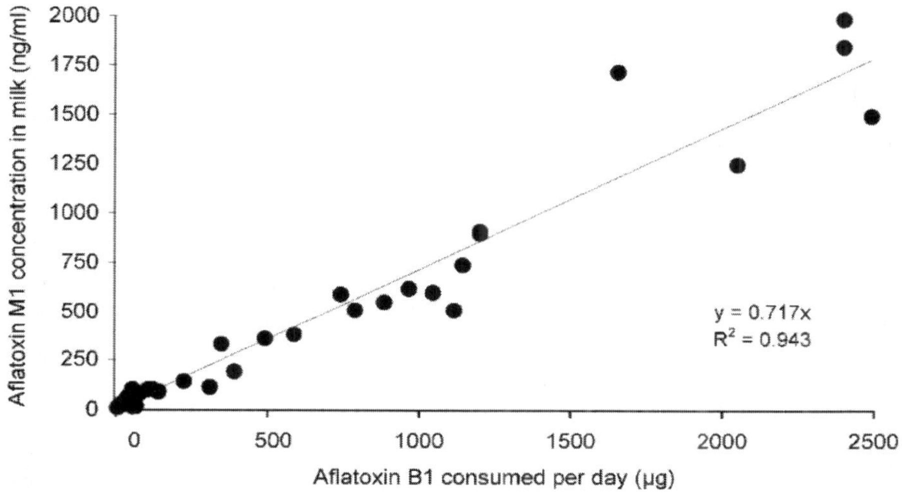

Fig.5.1: The relationship between AFM -1 in milk and amount of AFB – 1 consumed by the dairy cows

vi. From improper agricultural practices

Mould growth occur in feed ingredients by improper agricultural practices, like incorrect planting, cultivation and harvesting (Pre-harvest) and drying, storage of crops, transport and processing (Post-harvest). Mechanical damage occurs in grains while harvesting favours the mould growth. Piling or heaping the freshly harvested crops before drying favours fungal growth. In granary, storage container should be cleaned periodically and spilled grains should be collected and disposed off safely before mould growth begins.

vii. Indirect contamination due to combination of meteorological and environmental conditions while producing agricultural commodities

a. High temperature
b. Heavy rains
c. Chronic drought
d. Crop insect damage
e. Insect infestation

f. Poor fertility
g. Weed competition
h. High crop densities

B. Direct contamination

Occurrence of aflatoxin by fungus growth directly in milk and milk products also occurs. Occasionally other fungal species except *Aspergillus flavus* and *A. Parasiticus* accidentally contaminate cheese, which can produce aflatoxins like B1, B2, G1 and G2 (IDF, 1997).

Regulation of Aflatoxin M_1 in milk and dairy products

An acceptable level of aflatoxin M_1 in milk is 0.05 μg / Kg and not more than 20 μg / Kg in dairy cattle feeds as per EU limits (EU Regulation, 2001). The regulatory limit is set as 1.7% (range from 0.8 to 2.0%) of the concentration of aflatoxin in the dry matter consumed by the animal. For example dairy cattle consuming 30 μg / Kg of aflatoxin through feed will excrete 0.5 μg / Kg of AFM_1 in milk (EFSA, 2004).

The regulatory limits for aflatoxin in food vary from 0 to 50 μg / Kg (FAO, 2009). The levels of aflatoxin M_1 in milk should not exceed 0.5 μg / Kg as per United States regulations. However, the Codex Alimentarius set 50 ng/kg as the regulatory limit and for infant milk and follow-on milk, no more than 0.025 μg / Kg is allowed (EC, 2006).

Table 5.2: The maximum limits for mycotoxins prescribed under Food Safety and Standards Regulations 2011, (FSSR) by FSSAI

Commodity	μg / kg or ppb
Aflatoxin level	
Cereal and cereal by products	15
Pulses	15
Oilseed	
AFM – 1 level	
AFM-1 in milk	0.5
Ochratoxin level	
Wheat, rye, Barley	20
Deoxynivalenol level	
Wheat	1000

Table 5.3: Maximum acceptable levels of aflatoxin M-1 in milk and milk products in some countries

Region	Maximum acceptable level (ng/l)	Type
European Union	50	Milk
Austria	50	Milk
Argentina	50	Milk
Bulgaria	500	Milk
Germany	50	Milk
Australia	20	Children's milk
Sweden	50	Liquid milk products
Belgium	50	Milk
USA	50	Milk
Czech Republic	100	Children's milk
Serbia	500	Milk
Iran	50	Raw, pasteurized and Ultra-high temperature processing (UHT) milk
France	30	Children's milk <3 years
Turkey	50	Milk and milk products
Brazil	500	Milk

Table 5.4: The maximum limits for mycotoxins prescribed under Bureau of Indian Specification (BIS)

Commodity	µg / kg or ppb
Aflatoxin B-1 level	
Cattle feed (Type. I, II and III)	20
Broiler feed	20
Layer feed	20

Approaches to prevent AFM – 1 Contamination in Milk

To prevent fungal growth in feed and their hazardous toxin contaminating dairy products and environment, the following practices are recommended to reduce the AFM – 1 contamination in milk and milk products.

- Complete destruction of the contaminated products
- Detoxification or destruction of mycotoxin to the minimal level.

Mycotoxins in the contaminated feed should be detoxified by physical, chemical and biological methods for effective decontamination of mycotoxin.

A. Physical approaches

Mechanical separation, density segregation, colour sorting, removal of the fines or screenings significantly reduce the mycotoxin content of grains (Abdel-Wahhab and Kholif, 2010). Gamma irradiation is an effective method to detoxify the ochratoxin in feed (Refai *et al.*, 1996). The concentration of mycotoxin in the contaminated raw ingredients is diluted by blending to produce final feed below the critical level of mycotoxin (Schaafsma, 2002). Avoiding the usage of damaged portion of crops and removal of such damaged crop during harvesting may reduce the aflatoxin contamination in the grains during storage and transportation.

B. Physico chemical approaches

Using adsorbing agents to bind aflatoxin

Using adsorbing agents to bind aflatoxin in animal feed and reduce its distribution in animal tissues and milk. Aflatoxin content in milk can be reduced by the absorbents, because of its ability to bind to AFM-1 in a stable mode. Some of the adsorbents used as toxin binding agents are bentonite, vermiculite, hydrated sodium calcium aluminum silicate (HSCAS), and activated carbon (Asi *et al* ., 2012).

i. Bentonite

Bentonite is aluminum phyllosilicate clay. The negatively charged bentonite molecules pass through the gastrointestinal tract and bind to the positively charged toxin molecule. Then, the animal body can excrete the toxin filled clay through gut movements (Fowler and Bailey, 2015).

Two types of bentonite clay can be used as toxin binder. They are

1. Sodium-bentonite – It has electromagnetic properties. In the presence of water, it swells by six times and absorb the toxins (Jaynes *et al.*, 2007).
2. Calcium-bentonite – It is smaller in size and attracts the positively charged toxins by ions exchange resulting in absorbance of toxin molecule. These small particles can pass through the colon wall into the bloodstream where they get rid of toxins and leaves minerals behind (Iha *et al.*, 2013).

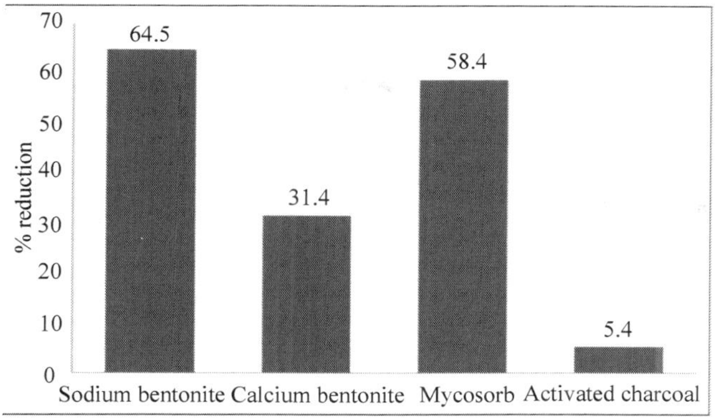

Fig. 5.2: Effectiveness of some compounds to reduce aflatoxin content in milk

ii. Hydrated sodium calcium aluminum silicate (HSCAS)

The hydrated HSCAS is a phyllosilicate clay with high affinity to aflatoxins and prevent aflatoxicosis in chickens, goats, cows and pigs (Abdel-Wahhab and Kholif, 2010).

iii. Activated carbon

Activated carbon is found to reduce the AFM-1 content in infected milk. Various research studies on mycotoxin indicated that supplementation of sodium bentonite and activated carbon (1%) has significantly reduced the aflatoxin M-1 content in milk without affecting the milk composition. Supplementation of activated carbon and HSCAS in aflatoxin contaminated feed of livestock reduces conversion of AFB -1 to AFM -1 in milk by 50 % and 36 % respectively. (Soha and Borji, 2007).

C. Chemical approaches

A wide variety of chemicals have been effectively used to detoxify aflatoxin. Chemicals such as acids, bases (Ammonia, Sodium hydroxide), oxidizing reagents (Hydrogen Peroxide, Ozone), reducing agents (Bisulphite, sugars), Chlorinating agents such as chlorine can be used to detoxify the mycotoxin. There are several risks associated with this treatment procedure and the end products produced must be removed before feeding. It is very difficult to detoxify the aflatoxin without affecting the nutritive value and palatability of the contaminated feed. It is expensive and time consuming and their effectiveness of treatment depends on the reaction time, temperature and moisture. Ammoniation treatment can diminish the aflatoxin in livestock feed by 79 – 90 %. Ammonia reacts with aflatoxin molecule by breaking oxygen bond (Phillips, 1999). Using H_2O_2 followed by heat treatment at 36° C for 30 minutes and 75°C for 15 seconds then boiling for 5 min could inactivate aflatoxin by 27.8% and 28.8 % respectively (Jouany, 2007). The addition of H_2O_2 or sodium hypochlorite in livestock feed and stored at room temperature for 7 days can destruct 62% and 82% of aflatoxin B-1 content in feed (Naeimipour *et al.,* 1998).

i. Using plant extracts to detoxify aflatoxin content in milk

Extracts of broccoli, garlic, cumin can be used as feed additives which effectively reduce the aflatoxin content in milk. Adding the extract of garlic, black cumin and carrot to milk in the ratio of 1:10 was significantly reduced the aflatoxin M-1 content in milk (Ayoub *et al*., 2011). Studies on effect of plant extracts on aflatoxin indicated that plant alkaloids like coumarins, flavonoid and curcuminoids inhibit biotransformation of aflatoxin to their active epoxide derivatives. Up to 2 % inclusion of turmeric concentration significantly decreases the aflatoxin content in milk (Naeimipour *et al.,* 2018).

ii. Oltipraz

Oltipraz, a new substituted dithiolthione which inhibits the aflatoxin B1 metabolism by inhibiting cytochrome P450 enzyme activities thereby reduction of aflatoxin M1 in the milk. Incubation of aflatoxin M1 and oltipraz with bovine hepatocytes resulted in less formation of aflatoxin M1 which indicates the effective inhibition of aflatoxin M-1 contamination of milk (Kuilman *et al*., 1998).

D. Biological approaches

i. Using probiotics to detoxify toxins in milk

The commercial bacterial strains used as probiotics such as Lactobacillus, Streptococcus, Pseudomonas, Bifidobacteria and Burkholderia can reduce AFM-1 contents in milk, and yogurt. It is found that *L. bulgaricus* has more binding ability than *S. thermophilus* (Ayoub *et al*., 2011). AFM-1level in milk reduced because of binding of AFM -1 to the cell wall components of probiotic microorganism. The enzymatic degradation of AFM-1 by Lactobacillus, Burkholderia and Pseudomonas species can also inhibit fungal growth and production of aflatoxins. Yeast like *Saccharomyces Kefir* has been used to eliminate high level of aflatoxin in milk. (Hwang *et al.,* 2005; El-kest *et al.,* 2015).

ii. Detoxification of mycotoxins by using microorganisms

Flavobacterium aurantiacum B- 184 have the ability to detoxify aflatoxins from milk, vegetable oil, maize, peanut and peanut milk (Line and Brackett, 1995). However, its usage in food industries is restricted because of occurrence of bright orange color pigmentation in food products. Impairing the nutritive value of the feedstuffs, changing the feed color or flavor and affecting the food safety are some of the negative effects encountered using certain microorganism for degradation (Shapira, 2004).

iii. Biodegradation of mycotoxins by microbial enzymes

To detoxify the mycotoxin, different microbial enzymes have been used by utilizing the metabolic potential of microorganisms (Asgher *et al.*, 2008). By using fermentation medium, selective microorganisms are cultured in huge tanks to produce enzymes as metabolites of microbial activity. These enzymes are extracted, purified and used for biodegrading mycotoxin in food industries.

Table 5.5: List of the microorganism and their mycotoxin degrading enzyme

S. No	Name of the microorganism	Type of enzyme produced	Type of aflatoxin detoxified	Reporting authors
1.	*Armillariella tabascens*	aflatoxin detoxifizyme (AFDF)	Aflatoxin	Liu *et al.*, (1998)
2.	Fungus *Peniophora* and *Pleurotus ostreatus*	laccase enzyme	Aflatoxin degradability 35 -40 %	Albert *et al.*, (2006)
3.	*Phaffia rhodozyma*	carboxypeptidase A	OTA degradation	Peteri *et al.*, 2007
4.	*A. niger*	carboxypeptidase A	OTA degradation	Abrunhosa and Armando, 2007

Different milk processing techniques to reduce the AFM – 1 content in milk

Heat processing techniques like pasteurization, boiling and ultra - high temperature processing techniques have no significant effect on reduction of AFM -1 concentration in milk. (Patel *et al.*, 1981; Henry *et al.*, 2001; Galvano *et al.*, 1996). However, Naeimipour, *et al.* (2018) reported 32 % of detoxification of AFM -1 in milk by heat processing techniques like pasteurization at 62°C for 30 minutes. Khoury *et al.* (2011) reported that Lactic acid bacteria such as *L. bulgaricus* and *Streptococcus thermophilus* were reduce the aflatoxin M-1 content in milk during yogurt processing.

6

Estimation of Mycotoxins

Mycotoxins are toxic secondary metabolites produced by different types of moulds which are present in soil, plant and feed ingredients. Ingestion of toxins will result in reduced growth and production performance due to reduced nutrient utilization, illness or death of animals. Analysing the presence of mycotoxin and its concentration in grain and feeds is necessary to eliminate the adverse health effects of mycotoxins in animals. Estimation of mycotoxin in feed ingredients is a challenging task because the concentration of toxin is at μg/kg or parts-per billion levels. At the same time, analysing inappropriate samples is a waste of resources. Mycotoxins are not evenly distributed in feeds or grains. If the specimen collected for analysis includes contaminated grain, the mycotoxin will be detected. If not, the mycotoxin will not be detected.

Sample collection for mycotoxin analysis

The objective of sample collection is to collect the specimen samples from as many parts of the feed lot as possible. The size of the collected specimen depends on the size of the load received. Sample collecting probes can be used to collect the samples from bags.

Table.6.1: Minimum number of bags required to collect sample from different feed lot

S. No	Load size	Sample size
1.	Up to 5 bags	All bags
2.	6 to 50	5 bags
3.	51 to 100	10% bags at random from different places
4.	101 to 300	5% bags but minimum 10 bags
5.	301 to 500	5% bags but minimum 15 bags

Mix the collected sample well and send it for analysis. If the sample is wet, keep the sample in the oven and send the sample at 13 % moisture level. Otherwise, in wet sample, fungi will grow during shipment. Mycotoxins are not significantly destroyed at 60 – 70°C while drying the samples in oven for moisture reduction. If wet sample cannot be dried, freeze the sample and send it at freezing temperature till it reaches the laboratory for mycotoxin analysis. Use paper or cloth bags than plastic bags for sample collection to prevent fungal growth during shipment.

In all experimental procedures followed in detecting the presence of mycotoxin either quantitatively or qualitatively, it involves the steps of extraction, clean up and separation of mycotoxin. Determination of mycotoxin must rely on the correct extraction and cleanup methods.

I. Extraction of mycotoxins from the samples

The purpose of extraction is to remove as much of the mycotoxin from the food matrix as possible into a solvent suitable for subsequent cleanup and determination. Foods are typically extracted with mixtures of water and relatively polar solvents (acetone, acetonitrile, ethyl acetate, methanol). Acetonitrile and methanol are the most common solvents used for extracting the major mycotoxins, with the exception of patulin for which ethyl acetate is preferred.

The extraction solvent is determined from the physical and chemical characteristics of the aflatoxin, the food/feed material, safety and the analytical procedures.

Chlorinated solvents (methylene chloride) are very efficient in extracting aflatoxins from maize. As methylene chloride is immiscible with water it cannot be used in aqueous analytical test (ELISAs)

Extraction can be done by

- High speed blending with solvent for few minutes
- Shaking with a solvent for 30 minutes or 2 hours

The solid samples are blend with the solvent and the liquid is separated by filtration. The extract is cleaned and toxins are isolated for quantification process.

II. Clean up procedure

As the mycotoxin is extracted from the solid into the solvent the impurities shall be removed and proceeded to the quantitative step. During cleaning process the toxin has to be extracted from the solvent as impurities will affect the sensitivity of the results. This step also concentrates the mycotoxin level before the estimation step. However, some techniques like ELISA don't require this cleanup step.

Glassware used for mycotoxin estimation should also be free of contamination, such as alkaline detergents, which can form salts with the compounds and result in lower detection rates. Several methods exist, for cleaning up mycotoxin samples, and some of those that are widely used have been described below.

a) Liquid – liquid extraction (LLE)

b) Solid phase extraction (SPE)

SPE are usually porous silica columns which have been designed to selectively absorb impurities or analyte. In many cases the impurities passes through the column and analyte is retained. The retained analyte can be removed with selective washing with rinse solution.

In other cases the columns are designed to trap impurities. The advantage of this type of extraction is that only extraction solvent is needed to purify the sample.

The following are the list of SPE columns used for mycotoxin clean up procedure.

- Anion exchange SPE
- Immuno affinity SPE

This is the state-of-the-art of mycotoxin cleanup and analysis procedure. In this method antibodies attached to inert material are used to bind the analyte with the impurities. The anlyte is then eluted through the column along with the solvent which denatures the antibody. The commercial immune affinity column available are aflatoxins, ochratoxin A, fumonisins, zearalenone, deoxynivalenol, and recently also for T-2 and HT-2 toxin. One advantage of immunoaffinity is the specificity of the column; it has specific interaction between the mycotoxin and the antibody.

- Solid phase micro extraction (SPME)
- Silica gel SPE

a. Liquid – liquid extraction

In liquid-liquid extraction, two solvents were used in which one is used to extract the toxin and other solvent is used to remove rest of the matrix. Solvents such as hexane and cyclohexane are to remove non-polar contaminants, e.g. lipids and cholesterol. This type of clean up procedure is effective for several toxins. Effectiveness of this procedure is dependent on type of toxin to be determined and the type of matrix being used.

Disadvantage of this procedure

1. It is time consuming procedure
2. Possible loss of sample by adsorption onto the glassware.

b. Solid phase extraction

The basic principle of SPE technology is a variation of chromatographic techniques based around small disposable cartridges which are stationary phase formed by using silica gel or bonded phases. The sample is loaded in one solvent, generally under reduced pressure, rinsed, where most of the contaminants are removed, and eluted in another solvent. This system can be used "on" and "off" line. These cartridges have a high capacity for binding of small molecules.

Types of stationary phase

Cartridges of stationary phase contain different bonding phases, ranging from silica gel, C-18 (octadecylsilane), florisil, phenyl, aminopropyl, ion exchange materials, both anionic and cationic, to affinity materials such as immunoadsorbents and molecular imprinted polymers (MIPs).

Advantages of SPE method over LLE

1. SPE procedure uses less solvent
2. It is a faster method
3. In addition to cleaning, this procedure is used to preconcentrate the samples resulting in better detection of toxin

Application of SPE method in extracting toxin

The following are the examples for successful extraction of toxin by using SPE.

Table 6.2: Different types of column used to extract mycotoxin

S. No	Column used	Extraction of toxin
1.	C – 18 Column	OTA extraction from wine sample
2.	SPME	OTA extraction from urine sample
3.	Immuno affinity SPE	OTA extraction
4.	Anion exchange SPE& Reverse phase C -18 cartridges	Fumonisin in plasma and urine samples
5.	C -18 RP	Aflatoxin in meat
6.	Silica gel SPE	Patulin
7.	C – 18 RP	Trichothecenes in grain

III. Separation methods

As per Pittet (2000), various methods and techniques followed to detect, identify and quantify mycotoxins are as follows.

Chromatographic techniques

a) Thin layer chromatography (TLC)

TLC is the first level of screening mycotoxin. It is relatively powerful tool to determine the presence of mixed mycotoxin in the sample.

In TLC the extract are spotted at the one end of the thin layer of silica gel coated on glass or aluminium plate. Samples are spotted along with the standards for comparison. The edges of the plate nearer to the solvent are placed in the suitable solvent. The solvent is absorbed by the silica matrix and travels upwards in vertical direction. During this process various compounds in the extract spotted are adsorbed based on their solubility. The compounds are deposited at different heights on the plate based on their properties. After the adsorption is completed they are removed from solvent, dried and viewed under UV lamp. Samples can be screened for mycotoxin based on visual estimation of fluorescence intensity under a UV lamp.

In extremely impure samples two-dimensional TLC can be utilized for estimation of mycotoxins. In such cases, a plate is developed with one solvent mixture in one direction, then rotated through 90° and run with a second solvent system. Often, unknown mycotoxins have been found on TLC plates which are usually ignored in other methods. Moreover, the identity of mycotoxin may be revealed on TLC, e.g. by spraying a suitable derivatization reagent lead to change in color.

A one-dimensional TLC method, combined with immuno affinity columns based clean-up is used to determine AFT in various food matrices (Stroka *et al.*, 2000). The AFT is quantified by densitometry. TLC analysis for detection of estrone, estradiol, diethylstilbestrol (DES), zearalanol (zeranol), zearalanone (ZON) and zearalenol (ZEL) has been reported by Medina and Schwartz (1992). TLC has been proved to be a cost efficient method of analysis for several mycotoxins with a fair amount of accuracy; further the chance of performing quantitative analysis makes it a generally excellent technique as systematic method.

b) High performance liquid chromatography (HPLC)

HPLC is the most widely used chromatographic technique used for mycotoxin analysis. Reference methods have been developed with high sensitivity and reasonably low level of detection.

HPLC separates toxins from the mixture (extract sample) by affinity difference between column and mobile solvent. The compound is eluted through the column and passed through the detector (fluorescence or UV), by which the toxins are quantitatively determine the toxin out of the injected sample.

In contrast to TLC where plates are used once, the life of HPLC analytical columns depends on the operating conditions. Injection of relatively "dirty" samples will drastically shorten column life and may lead to broader peaks if residues build up in the injector or column. Indeed, final extracts may still contain compounds not removed during cleanup that may or may not be related to the target mycotoxin. These substances may have retention times similar to the target analytes, thereby leading to false positives or mis-identification.

c) Gas chromatography (GC)

Gas chromatography is used for analysing some of the mycotoxins and in particular for the analysis of type-A trichothecenes (T-2 toxin, HT-2 toxin, neosolaniol and diacetoxyscirpenol) which cannot be detected in HPLC. In GC the components are separated using relative affinity for the column (Stationary column) and inert gas (mobile). Analytes eluted along with inert gases are detected either physically or chemically. Various detection system are done with coupling to GC, but in most cases electron-capture detection (ECD) and mass spectrometry (MS) have been employed. GC-ECD and GC-MS are highly sensitive methods that enable the simultaneous determination of several trichothecenes even in complex food matrices in the lower μg/kg range. Consequently, immunoaffinity and HPLC is now preferred to GC-ECD or GC-MS for the analysis of deoxynivalenol, T-2 and HT-2 toxins, which are the most prevalent trichothecenes and the only ones currently subjected to national and/or international regulations.

d) Capillary electrophoresis

Capillary electrophoresis (CE) is a chromatographic technique in which mycotoxins are separated from one another and from matrix components using electrical potential. In brief, a fused silica capillary (typical length 50 cm) is filled with an aqueous run buffer and an electric field is applied to the capillary. Separation is achieved by migration of charged particles in the run buffer. Cations migrate to the cathode and anions migrate to the anode under the influence of an electroosmotic flow. The analytes are then detected using fluorescence or UV absorbance.

The advantage in this technique is that there is less usage of solvent during the determinative step. As the buffers used are aqueous in nature the solvent utilization after extraction is eliminated.

e) Liquid chromatography coupled with mass spectrometry (LC- MS)

Liquid chromatography coupled with mass spectrometry (LC-MS) is a powerful tool for mycotoxin detection and identification, especially for the toxins with ultraviolet/visible (UV/VIS) absorbance or fluorescence, like the fumonisins and Alternaria toxins. However, the majority of LC-MS methods have been developed for the determination of trichothecene mycotoxins in various cereals.

Most of these methods employ either atmospheric pressure chemical ionization (APCI) or electrospray ionization (ESI) interfaces coupled with single or triple quadrupole mass spectrometers. Ion-trap instruments have also been utilized for trace level quantification of mycotoxins, but compared to triple quadrupole instruments, they suffer from certain drawbacks like lower limits of detection, poor calibration linearity, and lower measurement repeatability.

Liquid chromatography-atmospheric pressure chemical ionization tandem mass spectrometry (LC-APCI-MS/MS) is used for quantitative determination of the Fusarium mycotoxins ; deoxynivalenol, fumonisin B1 and zearalenone in maize. LC-ESI-MS/MS method is used for the determination of aflatoxins B1, B2, G1 and G2, ochratoxin A, deoxynivalenol, 3-acetyl deoxynivalenol, 15-acetyl deoxynivalenol, fumonisins B1 and B2, diacetoxyscirpenol, zearalenone, T-2 toxin, HT-2 toxin, roquefortine, and sterigmatocystin in single sample extracts.

Rapid screening methods

The majority of rapid screening methods rely on antibodies to detect mycotoxins (immunological assays).

f) Enzyme Linked Immuno Sorbent Assay (ELISA)

Sensitive microtiter plate immunoassays (ELISA format) are commercially available for a variety of mycotoxins including aflatoxins B, aflatoxin M1, ochratoxin A, fumonisins, zearalenone, deoxynivalenol, citrinin, and T-2 toxin.

Most of the ELISA kits are designed on competitive heterogeneous ELISA format. In these kits the sample competes with a labelled toxin for a limited number of antibody-binding sites. If more toxin is present in the sample there is less binding of the labeled toxin to the site and lower the signal generated from the essay. Presence of toxin is confirmed by the absence of the colour formed. The specificity of the result is reduced as any agent interfering the attachment of the labeled toxin is interpreted as aflatoxin. Usually structurally related mycotoxin as well as matrix constituents that is completely unrelated to mycotoxins but they interfere with conjugate attachment with antibody.

In other words, cross-reactivities and matrix dependence are the major drawbacks of ELISA methods, which can sometimes lead to a strong over estimation of mycotoxin contamination levels.

g) Dipsticks and lateral flow

In the dipstick immunoassay, instead of microtiter plates, carrier membranes (usually polyvinylidene difluoride, nylon or nitro-cellulose) are used to immobilize either the antibody or the antigen.

Lateral flow device contains an antibody coupled to a colored particle (such as colloidal gold or latex) which is deposited in a reservoir pad, and a target mycotoxin immobilized onto the membrane (the strip itself). When the sample solution is poured onto the reservoir pad or when the strip is placed in a vial containing the sample solution, the labelled antibody is solubilized and binds to the target mycotoxin, if present. Then this mycotoxin-antibody complex flows with the liquid sample laterally along the surface of the strip. When the complex passes over the zone where the target mycotoxin has been immobilized, nothing happens because the complex has no binding sites available. As a consequence, only one band will appear in the results window, indicating that the liquid flowed properly up the strip. In the case of a blank sample, the labelled antibody remains free and can bind to the mycotoxin immobilized on the test zone of the membrane, producing the appearance of a colored band on the strip. Therefore, the presence of two bands in the results window indicates a negative result. The smallest mycotoxin concentration that results in no color intensity is considered to be the visual detection limit

h) Molecular imprinted polymers

An interesting alternative to antibody based technologies is the development of non-biologically based binding elements like molecularly imprinted polymers (MIPs). Molecular imprinting is a process where functional and cross-linking monomers are co-polymerized in the presence of a target analyte (the imprint molecule), which acts as a molecular template. The functional monomers initially form a complex with the imprint molecule, and following polymerization, their functional groups are held in position by the highly cross linked polymeric structure. Subsequent removal (by liquid extraction) of the imprint molecule reveals binding sites that are complementary in size and shape to the analyte. In that way, a molecular memory is introduced into the polymer, which is now capable of selectively rebinding the analyte. The association between the imprint molecule and the monomers can be based on covalent, noncovalent or metal coordination interactions. The stability, ease of preparation and low cost of these materials make them particularly attractive.

i) Fluorescence polarization

Unlike most of the other immunoassays, the FP immunoassays are solution-phase assays: they can be conducted without the attachment of antibody to a solid surface. Fluorescence polarization detectors are indirectly measuring the rate of rotation of a fluorophore in solution. The rate of rotation is directly related to the size of molecules, with larger molecules rotating slower at a given temperature. With FP immunoassay a mycotoxin-fluorophore conjugate (tracer) is used. The tracer has a low molecular weight and rotates rapidly in solution. The addition of anti-toxin antibody results in the formation of an immune complex of the tracer with the antibody, effectively slowing the rate of rotation of the fluorophore and increasing the polarization.

The FP immunoassay therefore allows detection of low molecular weight materials in solution without requiring a step to separate the "free" and "antibodybound" toxin, which is a significant advantage over traditional ELISA techniques. However, the technique has limitations as well. Indeed, when compared with HPLC data, most of the FP experiments undertaken with various mycotoxins have shown a positive bias of 20 to 30%, which is resulting partly from known cross reactivities of the antibodies towards other fungal metabolites, and partly from matrix effects.

j) Biosensor

The development of biosensors for the rapid, reliable and low-cost determination of mycotoxins in foodstuffs has received considerable attention in recent years.

1. Surface plasmon resonance (SPR) is used to detect the change in mass during attachment of mycotoxin specific antibodies the surface of a sensor chip.

2. Fiber-optic probes can be used for continuous monitoring of toxin levels. The sensor uses the evanescent wave of light that form around the surface of an optical fiber. Antibodies attached to surface of fibre trap mycotoxin with the evanescent zone for easy detection.

7

Control Measures to Reduce Mycotoxins in Feed Ingredients and Crops

The economic loss in livestock arising due to mycotoxicosis is enormous apart from being a health risk. Indian economy is heavily affected by mycotoxins. It was estimated that 10 million dollars were lost in India's export within a decade due to groundnut contamination with mycotoxins (Vasanthi and Bhat, 1998). Many developing countries have realized that reducing mycotoxin contamination in foods will not only improve the health and production in animal, but also increase the raw material exports (international trade) to other countries. The following strategies are to be adhered strictly to reduce the mycotoxins contamination of crops in the field.

1. Early harvesting

Early harvesting reduces the fungal infection of crop in the field. Early harvesting and threshing of groundnuts results in lower aflatoxin levels and higher gross returns of 27% than in delayed harvesting (Rachaputi *et al.*, 2002).

2. Proper drying

Rapid drying of agricultural products to low moisture level within 24 - 48 hours would reduce the risk of fungal growth and subsequent aflatoxin production as it creates less favourable conditions for fungal growth and proliferation. Low moisture level should be maintained in all stages viz., storage, transportation and marketing.

3. Physical treatment

Traditional practices like sorting, winnowing, washing and crushing effectively removes mycotoxins. These processes separate the contaminated grain from the bulk.

4. Sanitation

Cleaning the godown / storage bin before loading new materials will reduce the aflatoxin contamination in the raw materials. Basic sanitation measures such as removal and destruction of debris from previous harvest would minimize the infestation of mould in the field.

5. Proper storage

Maintaining the moisture content of the feed at 10 % level is very important to preserve the quality of raw materials during storage. Proper storage measures like using insecticide to eliminate the insect infestation that increase the moisture content in the stored materials through respiration should be followed.

6. Insect management

The level of insect damage influences the extent of mycotoxins contamination. Insects carry spores of mycotoxins producing fungi from plant surfaces to the interior of the stalk or kernels or create infection wounds through their feeding habits (Munkvold, 2003). Therefore, proper management of insect pests through any appropriate control strategy would reduce mycotoxins contamination problem.

7. Using pesticide

Appropriate use of pesticides during the production process could help in minimizing the fungal infection or insect infestation of crops and consequently mycotoxin contamination. Fungicides such as itraconazole and amphotericin B effectively control aflatoxin producing *Aspergillus species* (Ni and Streett, 2005). Fumonisin contamination could be reduced by application of fungicides that have been used in control of Fusarium head blight such as prochloraz, propiconazole, epoxyconazole, tebuconazole, cyproconazole and azoxystrobin (Haidukowski *et al.*, 2004)

8. Using fungistatic agents

Fungistatic agents are low in molecular weight and their salts have been proven as a preserving agent for grains and animal feeds (e.g. propionic, formic and acetic acids).

Disadvantages of fungistatic agents are;

- Efficacy of fungistat is time dependent
- They are corrosive
- They destroy seed viability
- Acid treated grain is not accepted in commercial channals
- Direct inhalation or contact to human beings is harmful

9. Physical processing techniques for decontamination of mycotoxins

a. Heat

Aflatoxin are usually destroyed around 250°C as they are resistant to thermal inactivation. Therefore, any heat process techniques like roasting, cooking, frying and baking should reach the temperature range. The temperature used and time of exposure determines the destruction of mycotoxin.

b. Microwave

The principal of the microwave is to apply oscillating radio frequency or microwave field (500 MHz – 10 GHz) to sample thereby reorienting field direction of the water molecules, which creates intermolecular friction and heat generation. Depending on the microwave power and exposure time the Aflatoxin gets destroyed when exposed to microwave. As per the data 95 % of aflatoxin content in peanuts could be reduced with the exposure of microwave for 16 min 1.6 kW or a 5 min treatment at a power level of 3.2 kW (Luter *et al.*, 1982).

c. Irradiation

Irradiation has a multipurpose usage in agricultural produce. Radiation inhibits sprouting, delays ripening and eradicates all living factors responsible for food deterioration (insects, moulds and mites). The dosages required to degrade mycotoxin depends on the toxin concentration and the form of the toxin (e.g. pure toxin in powder or toxin in foods). Sometimes, irradiated fungi may produce large amounts of toxin. (Applegate and Chipley, 1974).

Adsorption of mycotoxins

Inclusion of aflatoxin binding materials in the diet is a novel approach used to prevent mould infestation in animals by binding the toxins in the gastrointestinal tract and decreasing the bioavailability and associated toxicity by altering toxin uptake into the blood and deposition in target organs. Hydrated sodium calcium aluminosilicate [HSCAS] adsorb aflatoxin B_1 with high affinity in milk, poultry, lambs and pigs. HSCAS decreases the level of AFM -1 in milk. Other binding agents like activated char coal, zeolite, bentonite, kaolin and montmorillonite can be used to adsorb aflatoxin, T-2 toxin, ochratoxin, DON, zearalenone and fumonisins.

As a conclusion, mycotoxin contamination in feed and fodder can be reduced by the following strategies:

1. With regard to feed ingredients

It must be dry

Oxygen free

Fermented or treated with mold growth inhibitors.

2. With regard to silage crops

Harvesting the crops at the appropriate moisture content

Packing and sealing the silo with suitable condition to exclude oxygen and allow the desirable microorganism growth for fermentaion.

Following the above said procedures are essential for reducing mycotoxin contamination in feeds and fodders.

8

Application of HACCP to Mycotoxins Control

Hazard Analysis Critical Control Points (HACCP) is an internationally recognized method of identifying and managing food safety related risk and, when central to an active food safety program, can provide customers, the public and regulatory agencies assurance that a food safety program is well managed. HACCP is a management system in which food safety is addressed through the analysis and control of biological, chemical, and physical hazards from raw material production, procurement and handling, to manufacturing, distribution and consumption of the finished product. (FAO, 2003)

Mycotoxin hazard analysis and identification of possible control measures

I. Hazard Analysis

a) Identification of mycotoxin hazard

For a given commodity system in a particular location, the HACCP team need to first consider which, if any, of the mycotoxins known to constitute a food safety hazard are likely to be present. Over 300 mycotoxins are known, but only a relatively few of these are widely accepted as presenting a significant food or animal feed safety risk.

The following mycotoxins have regulatory limits set by one or more countries: the aflatoxins (including aflatoxin M_1), ochratoxin A, zearalenone, patulin, ergot alkaloids, and deoxynivalenol. Guideline limits exist for fumonisin B_1 and regulatory limits are likely to be set in the near future. The regulatory limits are taken as the target levels and should be included in the Product Description table. Mycotoxin limits can also be set by the customer in specific contracts and it is possible that these may include mycotoxins not subject to regulatory limits.

The risk of a particular mycotoxin hazard should be estimated using well established data on the relative susceptibilities of commodities to given mycotoxins and the climatic conditions required for the mycotoxins to be produced. The EU has identified the following animal feed ingredients, and their products, as being highly susceptible to aflatoxin contamination: maize, groundnut cake, cottonseed cake, palm kernel cake and copra cake.

The EU has also identified the following foodstuffs as highly susceptible to aflatoxin contamination: dried figs and other dried fruit, groundnuts, pistachios and other edible nuts and cereals. These commodities are specified in the respective EC regulations (1525/98 amending regulation 194/97). Maize grown in temperate climates would be less likely to be contaminated with aflatoxin, but could be contaminated with trichothecene mycotoxins or fumonisin B_1. Although published mycotoxin survey data exists for many commodities, it is important that surveillance studies are performed if mycotoxin data is lacking for a particular commodity, or for production in a particular climatic zone.

b) Identification of steps in the Commodity Flow Diagram (CFD) where mycotoxin contamination is most likely to occur

Once the mycotoxin hazard(s) has been identified, each step in the CFD must be considered in turn and the likelihood of mycotoxin contamination occurring must be assessed. Usually published scientific data will be available to act as a guide, but it may be necessary to commission a study to determine, or confirm that the correct steps have been identified. The situation may change from year to year, and season to season, so there will need to be an element of mycotoxin surveillance in the HACCP plan.

An important fact to establish is whether pre-harvest contamination with mycotoxins is likely or whether contamination occurs primarily post-harvest. Mycotoxins produced by *Fusarium* spp, such as fumonisin B_1 are invariably produced pre-harvest, but climatic conditions affect the degree of blight and the resultant level of mycotoxin contamination. Aflatoxins can be produced both pre-harvest and post-harvest and climatic conditions can have a significant bearing: drought stress favours pre-harvest contamination, whereas post-harvest handling during the rainy season favours post-harvest aflatoxin contamination.

It is rarely possible to be certain that pre-harvest mycotoxin levels are below regulatory or target levels in the commodity system, so post-harvest mycotoxin control measures can often only prevent or reduce additional contamination, rather than prevent the hazard completely. Consequently it is often necessary to introduce a segregation step to remove any batches containing an unacceptable level of mycotoxin.

c) Possible Mycotoxin Control Measures

The most effective mycotoxin control measures is to dry the commodity such that the water activity (a_w) is too low to support mould growth and/or prevent mycotoxin production. To prevent the growth of most moulds the a_w needs to be £ 0.70, which translates to a moisture content of approximately 14% for maize and 7.0% for groundnuts at 20°C (the corresponding moisture content decreases as the temperature increases). Each toxigenic mould has its own minimum water activity for growth and mycotoxin production and these translate into moisture contents for each commodity. These moisture contents are termed 'safe' and would be the critical limit for the control measure.

It is important to specify target 'safe' moisture content with a maximum as well as an average value, e.g. 14% no part exceeding 15%. If only an average value is specified it may conceal a large range of moisture contents within the batch and the commodity would not be safe from mould growth and mycotoxin contamination. A drying process is required which dries evenly and the critical limits must be set bearing this in mind. Validation of such a CCP must involve moisture determination of multiple samples.

If the commodity is at 'unsafe' moisture content for longer than 48 hours, then mould can grow and mycotoxins be produced. Hence limiting the time that the commodity spends in the 'unsafe' moisture content window to less than 48 hours is a control measure. This explains why timely sun-drying can sometimes be safer than delayed mechanical drying. Two days on a drying floor with occasional turning can often achieve the target 'safe' moisture content, whereas a back-log at the mechanical drier can result in the critical limit of 48 hours not being met.

Once produced, it is not usually possible to remove mycotoxins, other than by physical separation (grading) techniques. To apply this type of control measure, representative samples of batches of commodity are collected and tested for selected mycotoxins. Only those batches containing less than the critical limit of mycotoxin, as specified in official regulations, are accepted. For some commodities, such as blanched groundnuts, colour sorters may be effective in rejecting individual high-aflatoxin nuts and accumulating low-aflatoxin nuts, and may be classified as a control measure.

There are a few examples where effective chemical detoxification is possible, such as ammoniation of certain animal feed ingredients and refining of vegetable oils. These are control measures that would also be suitable for application at a critical control point for aflatoxin, but only for the specified commodities.

It is essential that Good Agricultural Practice (GAP), Good Storage practice (GSP), and Good Mangement Practice (GMP) pre-requisites are in place, and simply ensuring that this is the case can significantly reduce the risk of the mycotoxin hazard. Examples of procedures which fall within the scope of these pre-requisites include: irrigation, insect control, use of resistant varieties, and use of pallets in store.

d) Determine Critical Control Points (CCPs)

Determination of CCPs can be achieved using a well designed decision tree, if necessary, to supplement the knowledge and experience of the HACCP team. Each step in the CFD is considered in turn, and the questions answered in sequence. It should be noted that it is necessary to be able to answer Yes to Question 1 (Do preventative control measures exist?) before a CCP can be established. The Codex 1997 definition of a control measure is any action and activity that can be used to prevent or eliminate a food safety hazard, or reduce it to an acceptable level.

There are commodity systems, such as the production of apple juice where control measures are possible at a number of steps, and each is capable of achieving a known percentage reduction in the level of mycotoxin. It is possible, therefore, to calculate the acceptable level of patulin at each step and perform validation. If the risk of the acceptable level of mycotoxin being exceeded is considered to be sufficiently low, then the HACCP team may determine each of the steps as CCPs.

e) Establish critical limits for each CCP

When the control measure is segregation based on mycotoxin analysis, then the critical limit will often be set at the acceptable level, which in turn will be set at, or below, the regulatory mycotoxin limit. Acceptable levels, and any associated critical limits, can sometimes be set higher than a regulatory limit, provided that a subsequent step can guarantee to attain the acceptable level of hazard in the final product.

For control measures that involve drying to a 'safe' moisture content, the parameter that will be measured, and for which critical limits will be set, will usually be parameters such as the temperature of the drier and the dwell time, e.g. for a continuous flow drier the critical limit for temperature could be 80 ± 2°C and the critical limit for dwell time could be 20 ± 1 minute.

Critical limits for chemical detoxification could be the temperature and pressure of the reaction vessel and the dwell time.

f) Establish a monitoring system for each CCP

The monitoring system must be a scheduled measurement, usually of a basic parameter such as temperature or time, to detect any deviation from the critical limits. When segregation of acceptable and unacceptable batches is required in the agricultural system, for example at a secondary trader, then rapid testing procedures are needed to test incoming batches.

A number of semi-quantitative immunoaffinity rapid test kits are available which work to a stated target level, eg. 5 or 20 μg/kg of the appropriate mycotoxin. Here the critical limit would normally be the presence or absence of a coloured derivative. More traditional mini-column and TLC dilution to extinction techniques can still be useful for segregation of batches at the factory gate, and for these the presence or absence of a blue fluorescent band or spot is the critical limit.

g) Establish a corrective action

There are two sorts of corrective action. The first is action to regain control. For instance if a critical limit for a moisture content is not attained, then the corrective action could be to check the specification of the drier and effect repairs, or perhaps to increase the temperature setting or the dwell time. The second type of corrective action is to isolate the product produced whilst the CCP was out of control and amend the product disposition, by either discarding or down-grading it, or re-processing it if this is appropriate.

h) Establish verification procedures

At regular, specified, intervals the complete HACCP plan should be verified by checking that the levels of mycotoxin in the final product are within acceptable levels. If this is found not to be the case, then immediately trouble-shooting should be carried out to identify the step at which the hazard has become out of control. Critical limits may need to be amended, or a new control measure may need to be validated and introduced. Similarly, if a review of deviations and product dispositions indicated an unacceptable degree of control at a particular CCP, then revisions will need to be made.

i) Establish documentation and record keeping

Standard HACCP documentation and record keeping is appropriate, but the complexity of the records should reflect the sophistication of the step in the commodity system.

II. Pre-requisite programmes

Pre-requisite programmes such as GAP, GMP and Good Hygienic Practice (GHP) must be working effectively within a commodity system before HACCP is applied. If these pre-requisite programmes are not functioning effectively then the introduction of HACCP will be complicated, resulting in a cumbersome, over-documented system.

a. Good Agricultural Practices

Primary Production

Primary food production should be managed to ensure that food is safe and wholesome for the consumer. Production will start on the farm, in the sea or lake or even within a forest. It is essential that certain ground rules are followed. Land used for crop or horticulture production should be fit for purpose and should not have previously been contaminated with heavy metals, industrial chemicals or environmental waste. Such hazards will be transferred into the food chain rendering the commodity unfit for human consumption. Farmers should control production so that contamination of the crop, proliferation of pests, and diseases of animals and plants, do not compromise food safety. GAP, including GHP where appropriate, should be adopted to make sure that the harvested commodity will not present a food hazard to the consumer.

Good Storage Practices (GSP) should be followed when the commodity is stored on the farm. As well as being covered in Food Hygiene Basic Texts (CODEX) there are also four ISO procedures that cover the storage of cereals and pulses (ISO 6322 series). GSP should also be followed for storage throughout the commodity system.

b. Good Manufacturing Practices

Establishment Design and Facilities

The structure and location of a processing plant needs to be considered in relation to the nature of operations and risks associated with them.

- Food premises should be designed to minimise possibilities of contamination of commodity or product.
- Design and layout should permit maintenance, cleaning and disinfection of the site to minimise airborne contamination.
- All surfaces that come into contact with food should be non toxic, as well as being easy to maintain and clean in order to prevent any additional contamination.
- Suitable facilities should exist for temperature and humidity control, when required.
- Effective measures should exist to prevent access by pests.

Control of Operation

Effective control measures should be in place to reduce the risk of contamination of the commodity or food supply such that it is safe and fit for the purpose:

- Adequate time, temperature or humidity controls
- Food grade packaging
- Potable water supplies
- Maintenance of equipment

Maintenance and Sanitation

Procedures and work instructions should exist to demonstrate an adequate level of maintenance of an establishment as well as efficient practices for cleaning, waste management and pest control. Overall, these operations will support the ongoing control of potential food hazards that may contaminate food.

Personnel Hygiene

Measures need to be in place to ensure that food handlers do not contaminate food. This objective can be attained by maintaining an appropriate level of personal cleanliness and following guidelines for personal hygiene.

Transportation

The method of transportation should be such that measures are taken to prevent any contamination or deterioration of the commodity. Commodities or product that need to be transported in certain environments should be appropriately controlled, e.g. chilled, frozen, or stored under specific humidity levels.

Containers and conveyors used for transporting food need to be maintained in good condition and be easy to clean. Containers used for bulk transfer should be designated and marked specifically for food use only.

Training

All food handlers should be trained in personal hygiene, as well as in the specific operation with which they are working, to a level commensurate with their duties. Food handlers should also be supervised by trained supervisors. An ongoing training programme for food handlers is paramount to the success of a Food Safety Management System

Product Information and Consumer Awareness

The end product should be accompanied by adequate information to ensure that personnel at the next stage in the food chain will handle, store, process, prepare and display the product safely. Since the consumer may be responsible for performing the ultimate control measure, the cooking of raw meat or fish. They should have all the relevant information required to carry out this step effectively. All batches of food should be easily identified, by a batch or lot number, to allow traceability of the commodity if required.

HACCP is a powerful tool with application to the control of mycotoxins in the commodity system. Undertaking a HACCP study focuses the thinking of everyone involved with the product on the details of the process, and promotes a greater awareness of safety issues. Implementation of a HACCP system is not an end in itself. The ongoing maintenance of the HACCP plan is where the benefit really lies.

References

Abdel-Wahhab, M. A. and Kholif, A. M. 2010. Mycotoxins in animal feeds and prevention strategies: a review. *Asian Journal of Animal Sciences*, **4**(3): 113-131

Abrunhosa, L. and V. Armando. 2007. Isolation and purification of an enzyme hydrolyzing ochratoxin A from Aspergillus niger. Biotechnol. Lett. 29: 1909-1914

Alberts, J. F., Engelbrecht. Y., Steyn. P.S., Holzapfel. W.H. and van Zyl. W.H. 2006. Biological degradation of aflatoxin B_1 by Rhodococcus erythropolis cultures. *Int. J. Food Microbiol.* **109**: 121-126.

Anfossi, L., Baggiani, C., Giovannoli, C. and Giraudi, G. 2010. Mycotoxins in food and feed: extraction, analysis and emerging technologies for rapid and on-field detection. *Recent Patents on Food, Nutrition & Agriculture*, **2**(2): 140–153. http://dx.doi.org/10.2174/2212798411002020140

Applegate, K. L. and Chipley, J. R. 1974. Effect of ^{60}Co GI on aflatoxin B_1 and B_2 production by *Aspergillus flavus*, Mycologia, **66**(3): 436–45

Asgher, M., M. Ashraf and R. L. Legge. 2008. Recent developments in biodegradation of industrial pollutants by white rot fungi and their enzyme system. *Biodegradation* **19**: 771-783.

Asi, M.R., Iqbal, S.Z., Arino, A. and Hussain, A. 2012. Effect of seasonal variations and lactation times on aflatoxin M_1 contamination in milk of different species from Punjab, *Pakistan. Food Control,* **25**: 34-8.

Ayoub, M., El-Far, A., Taha. N., Korshom, M., Mandour, A. and Abdel-Hamid, H. 2011. The biochemical protective role of some herbs against aflatoxicosis in ducklings: I. Turmeric. Lucrări Științ Univ Științ Agricole Med Veterinară Ser Zootehnie;55:150-9.

Bbosa, G.S.; Kitya, D.; Lubega, A.; Ogwal-Okeng, J.; Anokbonggo, W.W. and Kyegombe, D.B. (2013). Review of the biological and health effects of aflatoxins on body organs and body systems. In Aflatoxins—Recent Advances and Future Prospects; Razzaghi-Abyaneh, M., Ed.; InTech: Rijeka, Croatia, pp. 239–265, ISBN 978-953-51-0904-4

Bhat, R.V., Ramakrishna, Y., Beedu, S.R. and Munshi, K.L. 1989. Outbreak of trichothecene mycotoxicosis associated with consumption of mould damaged wheat products in Kashmir Valley, India. *Lancet* 1, 35–37

CAST, 2003. Mycotoxins — risks in plant, animal and human systems, Task Force Report, No. 139. Council for Agricultural Science and Technology, Ames, Iowa, pp. 1–191

Cheeke, P.R. 1998. Mycotoxins associated with forages. In: Cheeke, P.R. (Ed.), Natural Toxicants in Feeds, Forages, and Poisonous Plants. Interstate Publishers, Inc., Danville, IL, pp. 243–274.

Cheli, F., Campagnoli, A. and Dell'Orto, V. 2013. Fungal populations and mycotoxins in silages: from occurrence to analysis. Animal Feed Science and Technology, **183:** 1–16. doi:10.1016/j.anifeedsci.2013. 01.013

Colvin, B.M. and Harrison, L.R. 1992. Fumonisin-induced pulmonary edema and hydrothorax in swine. *Mycopathologia*, **117:** 79–82.

Creppy, E.E. 2002. Update of survey, regulation and toxic effects of mycotoxins in Europe. *Toxicology Letters*, **127**: 19 - 28.

Danicke, S., Gadeken, D., Ueberschar, K.H., Meyer, U. and Scholz, H. 2002. Effects of Fusarium toxin contaminated wheat and of a detoxifying agent on performance of growing bulls,on nutrient digestibility in wethers and on the carry over of zearalenone. Archiv fur Tierernahrung **56,** 245–261. doi:10.1080/00039420214347

Desjardins, A.E., Hohn, T.M. and McCormick, S.P. 1993. Trichothecene biosynthesis in Fusarium species: chemistry, genetics, and significance. *Microbiology and Molecular Biology Reviews,* Sep, **57**(3): 595-604.

Diaz, G.J. and Espitia, E. 2006. Occurrence of aflatoxin M_1 in retail milk samples from Bogota, Colombia. Food Additives & Contaminants, **23**(8): 811- 815. http:// dx.doi. org/10.1080/02652030600681617

Dien, H. and Schatzmayr, G. 2003. *Feed Mix*, Vol.**11**, No.1.

EC, European Commission. 2006. Commission regulation 1881/2006 of 19 December 2006 setting maximum levels for certain contaminants in foodstuffs. *Official Journal of the European Union, L* **364**, 5 – 24.

EFSA. 2004. Opinion on the scientific panel on contaminants in the food chain on a request from the commission related to aflatoxin B_1 as undesirable substance in animal feed. *The EFSA Journal,* **39**, 1 – 27.

El Marnissi, B., Belkhou, R., Morgavi, D.P., Bennani, L. and Boudra, H. 2012. Occurrence of aflatoxin M_1 in raw milk collected from traditional dairies in Morocco. Food and Chemical Toxicology: An International Journal Published for the British Industrial Biological Research Association, **50**(8), 2819 - 2821. http://dx.doi.org/ 10.1016/j. fct.2012.05.031.

El-kest, M.M., El-Hariri, M., Khafaga, N. and Refai, M.K. 2015. Studies on contamination of dairy products by aflatoxin M_1 and its control by probiotics. *J Glob Biosci*, **4**: 1294-312.

Engel, V.G. and Hagemeister, H. 1978. Untersuchungenueber den verblieb von aflatoxin B_1 im Verdaaundtarkt von Kuehen. Milchwissenschaft. *Milk Science International,* **33:** 21 –23.

EU Regulation 466/2001. (8 March 2001). Setting maximum levels for certain contaminants in foodstuff. *Official J. of European Commission,* **L077**, 11 - 12.

FAO. 2003. Manual on the Application of the HACCP System in Mycotoxin Prevention and Control, Rome, Italy.

FAO. 2004. Food and Nutrition Paper No. 81, 2004. Worldwide Regulations for Mycotoxins in Food and Feed in 2003. 180 pages.

FAO/WHO. 2009. Evaluation of certain food additives. Sixty-ninth report of the Joint FAO/ WHO Expert Committee on food additives. Geneva: World Health Organization (WHO Technical Report Series, No. 952 http://whqlibdoc.who.int/trs/WHO_TRS_952_eng.pdf

FDA. 1994. Food Labeling: Reference Daily Intakes. *Fed. Regist.* **59** (2), 427 -432.

Fink-Gremmels, J. 2008. Mycotoxins in cattle feeds and carry-over to dairy milk: a review. Food Additives & Contaminants: Part A. Chemistry, Analysis, Control, Exposure & Risk Assessment 25, 172–180. doi:10.1080/02652030701823142

Fowler, J., Li, W. and Bailey, C. 2015. Effects of a calcium bentonite clay in diets containing aflatoxin when measuring liver residues of aflatoxin B_1 in starter broiler chicks. *Toxins (Basel)*; **7**: 3455-64.

Galvano, F., Galofaro, V. and Galvano, G. 1996. Occurrence and stability of aflatoxin M_1 in milk and milk products: a worldwide review. *Journal of Food Protection*; **59**: 1079 - 1090.

Galvano, F., Galofaro, V., Ritieni, A., Bognanno, M., De Angelis, A., Galvano, G. 2001. Survey of the occurrence of aflatoxin M_1 in dairy products marketed in Italy: Second year of observation. *Food Addit Contam*; **18**: 644-6.

Haidukowski, M., Pascale, M., Perrone, G., Pancaldi, D., Campagna, C. and Visconti, A. 2004. Effect of fungicides on the development of Fusarium head blight, yield and deoxynivalenol accumulation in wheat inoculated under field conditions with Fusarium graminearum and Fusarium culmorum. *J. Sci., Food Agric*, **85:** 191–198.

Halasz, A., Latsztity, R., Abonyi, T. and Bata, A. 2009. Decontamination of Mycotoxin-containing food and feed by biodegradation. *Food Reviews International,* **25**: 284-298

Henry, S.H., Whitaker, T., Rabbani, I., Bowers, J., Park, D., Price, W. and Bosch, F.X. 2001. Aflatoxin M_1. Joint FAO / WHO Expert Committee o Food additives (JECFA); 47.

Hovermale, J.T. and Craig, A.M. 2001. Correlation of ergovaline and lolitrem B levels in endophyte-infected perennial ryegrass (*Lolium perenne*). *Journal of Veterinary Diagnostic Investigation,* **13:** 323–327.

Howell, V. Mary. 1982. Moulds and mycotoxins in animal feedstuffs. In: Haresign, W, Recent advances in animal nutrition - 1982. Butterworth publication, pp. 3 – 20.

Huszenicza, G., Fekete, S., Szigeti, G., Kulcsar, M., Febel, H., Kellems, R.O., Nagy, P., Cseh, S., Veresegyhazy, T. and Hullar, I. 2000. Ovarian consequences of low dose peroral Fusarium (T-2) toxin in a ewe and heifer model. *Theriogenology*, **53:** 1631–1639.

Hwang, K.T., Lee, W., Kim, G.Y., Lee, S.K., Lee, J. and Jun, W. 2005. The binding of aflatoxin B_1 modulates the adhesion properties of Lactobacillus casei KCTC 3260 to a HT29 colon cancer cell line. *Food Sci Biotechnol*; **14**: 866-70.

IARC. 2002. IARC monographs on the evaluation of carcinogenic risks to humans. In Traditional herbal medicines, some mycotoxins, napthalene and styrene (Vol. 82). Lyon: IARC Press.

IDF. 1997, Residues and Contaminants in Milk and Milk Products, International Dairy Federation, Brussels, pp 79 to 88.

Iha, M.H., Barbosa, C.B., Okada, I.A. and Trucksess, M.W. 2013. Aflatoxin M_1 in milk and distribution and stability of aflatoxin M_1 during production and storage of yoghurt and cheese. *Food Control*, **29**: 1-6.

Iqbal, S. Z., Asi, M. R. and Jinap, S. 2014. A survey of aflatoxin M_1 contamination in milk from urban and rural farm houses of Punjab, Pakistan. *Food Additives and Contaminants Part-B*, **7**(1): 17 -20.

Iqbal, S. Z., Paterson, R. R. M., Bhatti, I. A. and Asi, M. R. 2010. Survey of aflatoxins in chilies from Pakistan produced in rural, semi-rural and urban environments. *Food Additive and Contaminants Part-B*, **3**(4): 268 – 274.

Iqbal, S.Z., Jinap, S., Pirouz, A.A. and Ahmad Faizal, A.R. 2015. Aflatoxin M_1 in milk and dairy products, occurrence and recent challenges: A review. *Trends in Food Science & Technology,* **46**: 110 -119. 10.1016/j.tifs.2015.08.005.

Jaynes, W., Zartman, R. and Hudnall, W. 2007. Aflatoxin B_1 adsorption by clays from water and corn meal. *Appl Clay Sci* ; **36**: 197-205.

Jouany, J.P. 2007. Methods for preventing, decontaminating and minimizing the toxicity of mycotoxins in feeds. *Anim Feed Sci Technol*, **137**: 342-62

Kennedy, D.G., Hewitt, S.A., Mc Evoy, J.D., Currie, J.W., Cannavan, A., Blanchflower, W.J. and Elliot, C.T. 1998. Zeranol is formed from Fusarium spp. toxins in cattle *in vivo. Food Addit. Contam.***15**(4): 393-400.

Khoury, A., EL Atoui, A. and Yaghi, J. 2011. Analysis of aflatoxin M_1 in milk and yogurt and AFM_1 reduction by lactic acid bacteria used in Lebanese industry. *Feed Control*; **22:** 1695 -1699.

Kiessling, K.H., Pettersson, H., Sandholm, K. and Olsen, M.O.N.I.C.A., 1984. Metabolism of aflatoxin, ochratoxin, zearalenone, and three trichothecenes by intact rumen fluid, rumen protozoa, and rumen bacteria. *Applied and Environmental Microbiology*, **47**(5), pp.1070-1073.

Kuilman, M.E.M., Maas, R.F.M., Judah, D.J. and Gremmels, J. 1998. Bovine hepatic metabolism of aflatoxin B_1. *J. Agric. Food. Chem.*, **46**: 2707-2713.

Laan, T., Bull, S., Pirie, R. and Fink-Gremmels, J. 2006. The role of alveolar macrophages in the pathogenesis of recurrent airway obstruction in horses. *Journal of Veterinary Internal Medicine*, **20**: 167–174.

Line, J.E. and Brackett, R.E. 1995. Factors affecting aflatoxin B_1 removal by *Flavobacterium aurantiacum*. *J. Food Prot.*, **58**: 91- 94.

Liu Yang. 2010. Effects of feed types on OTA biodegradation by Korean native goats. Masters' Thesis, Seoul National University.

Liu, D.L., Yao, D.S., Liang, R., Ma, L., Cheng, W.Q. and Gu, L.Q. 1998. Detoxification of aflatoxin B_1 by enzymes isolated from Armillariella tabescens. *Food. Chem. Toxicol.* **36**: 563-574.

Luongo, L., Galli, M., Corazza, L., Meekes, E., Haas, L., Plas, L.C. and Kohl, J. 2005. Potential of fungal antagonists for bio-control of Fusarium spp. in wheat and maize through competition in crop debris. *Biocontrol Sci. Technol.* **15**: 229–242.

Luter, L., Wyslouzil, W. and Kashyap, S.C. 1982. The destruction of aflatoxin in peanuts by microwave roasting, *Can. Inst. Food Sci. Technol. J.,* **15**(3): 236–8.

Marasas, W.F.O., Nelson, P.E. and Toussoun, T.A. 1984. Toxigenic Fusarium species: identity and mycotoxicology. The Pennsylvania State University Press, University Park, Pa.

Marasas, W.F.O., Kellerman, T.S., Gelderblom, W.C.A., Coetzer, J.A.W., Thiel, P.G and van der Lugt, J.J. 1988. Leukoenchapalomalacia in a horse induced by fumonisin B_1, isolated from *Fusarium moniliforme*. *Onedersteport Journal of Veterinary Research,* **55:** 197–203.

Marchese, S., Polo, A., Ariano, A., Velotto, S., Costantini, S. and Severino, L. 2018. Aflatoxin B_1 and M_1: Biological properties and their involvement in cancer development. *Toxins*, **10**(6): p.214

Marczuk, J., Obremski, K., Lutnicki, K., Gajecka, M. and Gajecki, M. 2012. Zearalenone and deoxynivalenol mycotoxicosis in dairy cattle herds. *Polish Journal of Veterinary Sciences*, **15**: 365–372. Doi:10.2478/ v10181-012-0055-x.

Marth, E.H. and Steele, J.L. 1998. Applied Dairy Microbiology, Marcel Dekker Inc. New York, pp 280 to 285.

May, H.D., Wu, Q. and Blake, C.K. 2000. Effects of the Fusarium spp. mycotoxins fusaric acid and deoxynivalenol on the growth of *Ruminococcus albus* and *Methanobrevibacter ruminantium*. *Canadian Journal of Microbiology*, **46:** 692–699. doi:10.1139/cjm-46-8-692.

Medina, M.B. and Schwartz, D.P. 1992. *J. Chromatogr.*, 581:119

Morgavi, D., Boudra, H., Jouany, J. and Graviou, D. 2003. Prevention of patulin toxicity on rumen microbial fermentation by SH-containing reducing agents. *Journal of Agriculture and Food Chemistry*, 51: 6906– 6910

Munkvold, G.P. 2003. Cultural and genetic approaches to managing mycotoxins in maize. *Ann. Rev. Phytopathol.*, **41:** 99–116.

Naeimipour, F., Aghajani, J., Kojuri, S.A. and Ayoubi, S. 2018. Useful approaches for reducing aflatoxin M_1 content in milk and dairy products. *Biomedical and Biotechnology Research Journal (BBRJ)*, **2**(2): p.94.

Nanthini, A.R. and Radhakrishnan, L. 2016. Incidence of Multi mycotoxin in different agro commodities used for preparing livestock feeds, *The Indian Veterinary Journal*, **93**(01): P. No. 20 – 22

Neal, G.E., Eaton, D.L., Judah, D.J. and Verma, A. 1998. Metabolism and toxicity of aflatoxins M_1 and B_1 in human-derived in vitro systems. *Toxicol. Appl. Pharmacol.*, **151**: 152–158.

Ni, X. and Streett, D.A. 2005. Modulation of water activity on fungicide effect on *Aspergillus niger* growth in Sabouraud dextrose agar medium. *Lett. Appl. Microbiol.* **41**: 428–433.

Niyo, K.A., Richard, J.L. and Tiffany, L.H. 1988. Effect of T-2 mycotoxin ingestion on phagocytosis of Aspergillus fumigatus conidia by rabbit alveolar macrophages and on hematologic, serum biochemical, and pathologic changes in rabbits. *American Journal of Veterinary Research*, **49:** 1766–1773.

Patel, P.M., Netke, S.P., Gupta, D.S. and Dabadghao, A.K. 1981. Note on the effect of processing milk into khoa on aflatoxin M_1 content. *Indian Journal of Animal Sciences,* **51:** 791 – 792.

Pestka, J.J. and Bondy, G.S. 1994. Immunotoxic effects of mycotoxins. In: Miller, J.D., Trenholm, H.L. (Eds.), Mycotoxins in Grain-Compounds other than Aflatoxin. Eagan Press, St. Paul, pp. 339–358.

Peteri, Z., Terenb, J., Vagvo lgyia, C. and Varga, J. 2007. Ochratoxin degradation and adsorption caused by astaxanthin producing yeasts. *Food Microbiol.***24**: 205-221.

Pettersson, H. 2004. Controlling mycotoxins in animal feed, In: Magan. N and Olsen. M (Eds.), Mycotoxins in food; Detection and control, CRC Press, Woodhead Publishing Limited, Cambridge England, pp: 262 – 304.

Pfohl-Leszkowicz, A., Petkova-Bocharova, T., Chernozemsky, I.N. and Castegnaro, M., 2002. Balkan endemic nephropathy and associated uringary tract tumours: a review on aetiological causes and the potential role of mycotoxins. *Food Additives and Contaminants*, **19:** 282–302.

Phillips, T.D. 1999. Dietary clay in the chemoprevention of aflatoxininduced disease. *Toxicol Sci.*, **52**: 118-26.

Pittet A. Natural Occurrence of Mycotoxins in Foods and Feeds: a Decade in Review. In: Mycotoxins and Phycotoxins in Perspective at the Turn of the Millennium (Proceedings of the Xth International IUPAC Symposium on Mycotoxins and Phycotoxins, 21–25 May, 2000, Guaruja, Brazil). Edited by W.J. de Koe et al., Publ. W.J. de Koe, Hazekamp 2, 6707 HG Wageningen (The Netherlands), 2001. Chapter 6, pp. 153–172.

Prelusky, D.B., Rotter, B.A., Rotter, R.G., 1994. Toxicology of mycotoxins. In: Miller, J.D., Trenholm, H.L. (Eds.), Mycotoxins in Grain-Compounds other than Aflatoxin. Eagan Press, St. Paul, pp. 359–403.

Rachaputi, N.R., Wright, G.C. and Kroschi, S. 2002. Management practices to minimise pre-harvest aflatoxin contamination in Australian groundnuts. *Austr. J. Exp. Agric*. **42:** 595–605.

Refai, M.K., Aziz, N.A., El – Far, F. and Hassan, A.A. 1996. Detection of ochratoxin produced by *Aspergillus ochraceus* in feedstuffs and its control by β – radiation. *Applied Radiat. Isot.*,**47**: 617 – 621.

Richard, J.L. 1991. Mycotoxins as immunomodulators in animal systems. In: Bray, G.A., Ryan, D.H. (Eds.), Mycotoxins, Cancer, and Health, Pennington Center Nutrition Series. Louisiana State University Press, Baton Rouge, Louisiana, pp. 197–220.

Richard, J.L., 1998. Mycotoxins, toxicity and metabolism in animals - a systems approach overview. In: Miraglia, M., van Egmond, H.P., Brera, C., Gilbert, J. (Eds.), Mycotoxins and Phycotoxins - *Developments in Chemistry, Toxicology and Food Safety*. Alaken, Inc., Fort Collins, pp. 363–397

Richard, J.L., 2000. Mycotoxins—an overview. In: Richard, J.L. (Ed.), Romer Labs' Guide to Mycotoxins, vol. 1, pp. 1–48.

Richard, J.L., Meerdink, G., Maragos, C.M., Tumblesom, M., Bordson, G., Rice, L.G. and Ross, P.F. 1996. Absence of detectable fumonisins in milk of cows fed Fusarium proliferatum (Matsushima) Nirenberg culture material. *Mycopathologia* **133**, 123–126.

Richard, J.L., Plattner, R.D., May, J. and Liska, S.L. 1999. The occurrence of ochratoxin A in dust collected from a problem household. *Mycopathologia*, **146**: 99–103

Russell, L., Cox, D.F., Larsen, G., Bodwell, K. and Nelson, C.E. 1991. Incidence of molds and mycotoxins in commercial animal feed mills in seven midwestern states 1988–1989. *J. Anim. Sci.,* **69**: 5–12.

Salunkhe, D.K., Adsule, R.N. and Padule, D.N. 1987. Aflatoxins in foods and feeds, Metropolitan, Book Co. Pvt. Ltd., New Delhi, India, p.18.

Schaafsma, A.W. 2002. Economic changes imposed by mycotoxins in food grains: case study of deoxynivalenol in winter wheat. In Mycotoxins and food safety (pp. 271-276). Springer, Boston, MA.

Schatzmayr, G., Heidler, D., Fuchs, E., Loibner, A.P., Braun, R. and Binder, E.M. 2002. Evidence of ochratoxin A-detoxification activity of rumen fluid, intestinal fluid and soil samples as well as isolation of relevant microorganisms from these environments. *Mycotoxin Res.* **18A**:183-187.

Schatzmayr, G., Zehner, F., Taubel, M., Schatzmayr, D., Klimitsch, A., Loibner, A.P. and Binder, E.M. 2006. Microbiologicals for deactivating mycotoxins. *Mol. Nutr. Food Res.* **50**: 543-551.

Seeling, K., Lebzien, P., Danicke, S., Spilke, J., Sudekum, K.H. and Flachowsky, G. 2006. Effects of level of feed intake and Fusarium toxin-contaminated wheat on rumen fermentation as well as on blood and milk parameters in cows. *Journal of Animal Physiology and Animal Nutrition,* **90:** 103–115. doi:10.1111/j.1439-0396.2005.00570.x

Shapira, R. 2004. Detection and control. In Qinghua Wu, Alena Jezkova, Zonghui Yuan, Lucie Pavlikova, Vlastimil Dohna,and Kamil Biological degradation of aflatoxins. *Drug Metab. Rev.* **41**(1): 1-7.

Skaug, MA., Wignand, E. and Stormer, F.C. 2001. Ochratoxin A in airborne dust and fungal conidia. *Mycopathologia,* **151**: 93 – 98

Soha, A. and Borji, M. 2007. Reductions of aflatoxin M_1 in milk utilizing some chemisorption compounds and study their effects on milk composition. *Pajouhesh Sazandegi,* **1**: 19-26.

Sreemannarayana, O., Frohlich, A.A., Vitti, T.G., Marquardt, R.R. and Abramson, D. 1988. Studies of tolerance and disposition of ochratoxin A in young calves. *J. Anim. Sci.***66**: 1703-1711.

Stegelmeier, B.L., James, L.F., Panter, K.E., Ralphs, M.H., Gardner, D.R., Molyneux, R.J., Pfister, J.A. 1999. The pathogenesis and toxicokinetics of locoweed (Astralagus and Oxytropis spp) poisoning in livestock. *Journal of Natural Toxins,* **8:** 35–45.

Stroka, J., Otterdijk, R.V. and Anklam, E. 2000. *J. Chromatogr.* A 904: 251.

Sweeney, M.J. and Dobson, A.D.W. 1998. Mycotoxin production by Aspergillus, Fusarium and Penicillium species. *International Journal of Food Microbiology,* **43:** 141 -158.

Upadhaya, S.D., Park, M.A. and Ha, J.K. 2010. Mycotoxins and their biotransformation in the rumen: a review. *Asian–Australasian Journal of Animal Science,* **23:** 1250–1260.

Van Egmond, H.P. 1989. Mycotoxins in Dairy Products, Elsevier Applied Science, England

Vasanthi, S. and Bhat, R.V. 1998. Mycotoxins in foods-occurrence, health and economic significance and food control measures. *Ind. J. Med. Res.,* **108:** 212–224.

Veldman, A., Meijs, J., Borggreve, G. and Heeres-van der Tol, J. 1992. Carry-over of aflatoxin from cows' food to milk. *Anim. Sci.,***55:** 163–168.

Verma, R.J. 2004. Aflatoxin Cause DNA Damage. *Int. J. Hum. Genet.,* **4:** 231–236.

WHO Food Additives Series: 44, 2000. Zearalenone, 53rd meeting of JECFA. (http://www.inchem.org./documents/jecfa/jecmono/v44jec14.htm).

Wild, C.P. and Turner, P.C. 2002. The toxicology of aflatoxins as a basis for public health decisions. *Mutagenesis,***17:** 471–481